Acute Surgical Topics

Constantine P. Spanos

Acute Surgical Topics

An Infographic Guide

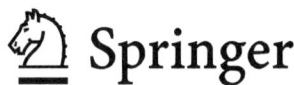 Springer

Constantine P. Spanos
1st Department of Surgery
Aristotelian University School of Medicine
Thessaloniki
Greece

ISBN 978-3-030-68699-4   ISBN 978-3-030-68700-7   (eBook)
https://doi.org/10.1007/978-3-030-68700-7

This Springer imprint is published by the registered company Springer Nature Switzerland AG
The registered company address is: Gewerbestrasse 11, 6330 Cham, Switzerland

To my wife Evangelia, and my daughters Marianna, Fotini, and Athena, for all their love and support.

Contents

- Labs and tests are a significant component of evaluation prior to surgery. Unnecessary labs and tests lead to increased costs; occasionally they lead to more unnecessary tests. A careful history, physical exam, and thorough review of systems will determine the appropriate preoperative laboratory interventions needed.
- A healthy patient undergoing surgery has no symptoms, comorbidities and can perform at least four metabolic equivalents (MET) of activity without symptoms. No preoperative labs are needed, regardless of age.
- Examples of METs:
  - Dressing up, eating, use of toilet alone = 1 MET
  - Walking up one flight of steps or hill or level ground walking (up to 6 km/h) = 4 METs
  - Heavy work around the house (scrubbing floors, lifting furniture, walking up two flights of stairs) = 4–10 METs
  - Participation in strenuous sports activities (swimming, tennis, football, basketball, skiing): >10 METs
- Patients with a history of seizures on antiseizure medication are at risk when electrolyte abnormalities exist. These may lower the seizure threshold. A basic metabolic panel (BMP) is obtained. BMP = Na^+, K^+, Blood urea nitrogen (BUN), creatinine.
- Strokes are associated with atrial fibrillation and atherosclerosis. In these patients, a complete blood count, BMP, and ECG are obtained.
- Cardiovascular disease includes coronary artery disease, peripheral vascular disease, carotid artery disease, and abdominal aortic aneurysmal disease. In these patients a CBC, BMP, and electrocardiogram are obtained.
- Patients with pulmonary disorders and a recent change in symptoms should get a chest X-ray. Patients with COPD and reactive airway disease are evaluated with spirometry and arterial blood gasses (ABGs). A $paCO_2 > 45$ mmHg is predictive of postoperative pulmonary complications.

Airflow optimization and infection prevention in patients with severe pulmonary disease includes:
  - Smoking cessation 8 weeks prior to operation
  - Bronchodilators
  - Inhaled steroids
  - Antibiotics
  - Incentive spirometry
- Liver disease is a risk factor for perioperative bleeding, infection, and wound complications. A CBC, BMP, AST/ALT, PT, PTT/INR are obtained.
- Diabetic patients are at risk for perioperative complications. Optimization of HgbA1c (glycosylated hemoglobin) may lead to better surgical outcomes and should be obtained preoperatively.
- Malnutrition may lead to anemia, electrolyte abnormalities, and coagulation defects. A CBC, BMP, PT, PTT/INR, and serum albumin are obtained.
- Renal disease is associated with anemia, electrolyte abnormalities, perioperative arrhythmias, bleeding, and anesthetic complications. A CBC, BMP, and ECG are obtained.
- Hematological diseases may lead to anemia, thrombocytopenia, and bleeding tendency. A CBC, BMP, PT, PTT/INR are obtained.
- Review of medications is extremely important regarding their effect on bleeding risk, electrolyte abnormalities, and pharmacokinetics with organ dysfunction. Below are examples of drugs and labs obtained:
  - Anticoagulants(coumadin): PT, PTT/INR
  - Antiplatelet drugs (aspirin, clopidogrel): CBC
  - Diuretics: BMP
  - Novel direct anticoagulants: BUN/creatinine
- Smokers should quit (ideally) or stop smoking 8 weeks prior to surgery. Patients consuming alcohol should get AST/ALT, PT, PTT/INR if there is suspicion of liver disease.

C. P. Spanos, *Acute Surgical Topics*, https://doi.org/10.1007/978-3-030-68700-7_1

Preoperative Labs and Tests

Unnecessary tests lead to increased costs; a careful history/physical exam and thorough review of systems will determine appropriate preoperative labs and tests needed

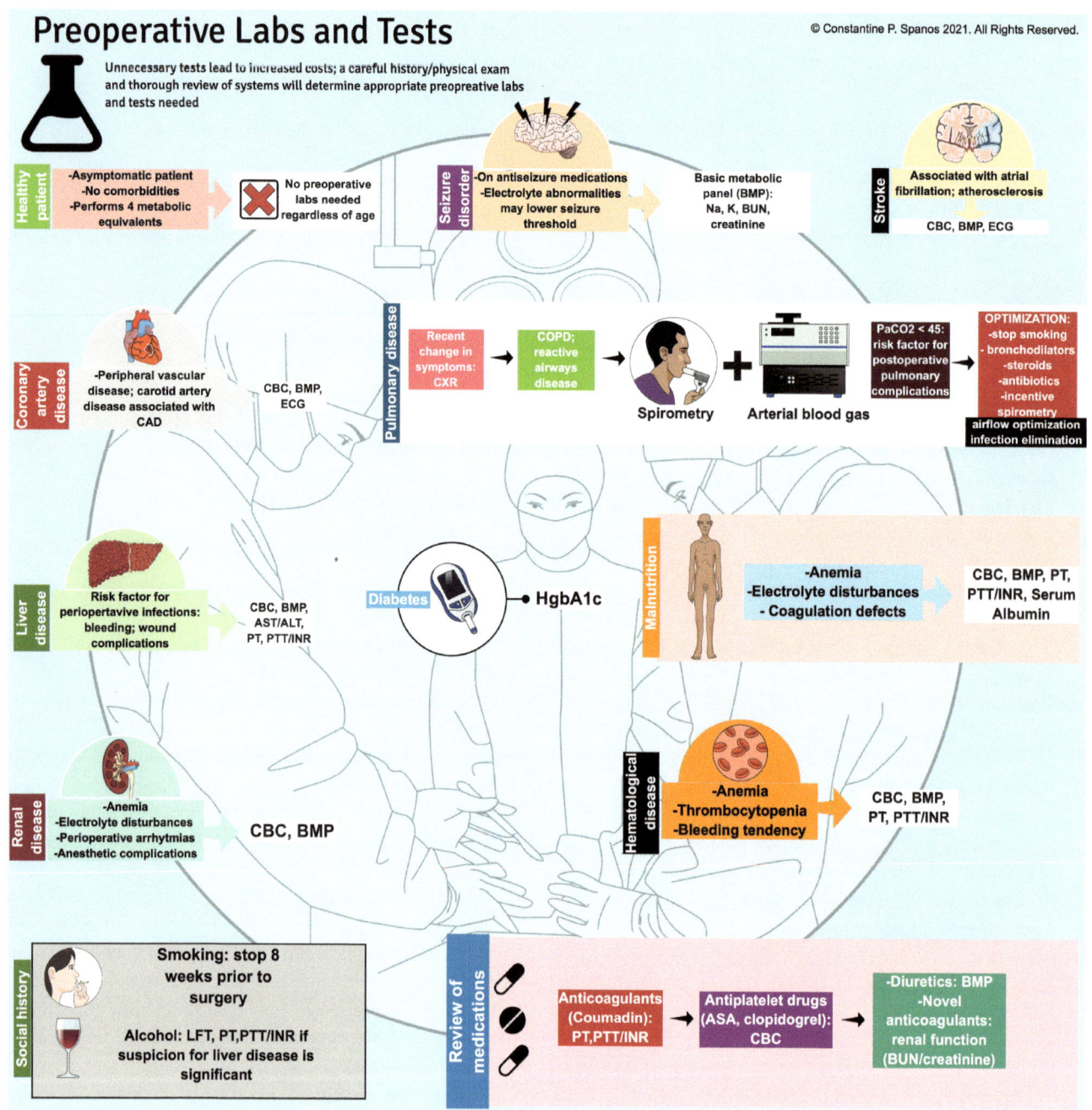

Further Reading

Benarroch-Gampel J, Sheffield KM, Duncan CB, et al. Preoperative laboratory testing in patients undergoing elective, low-risk ambulatory surgery. Ann Surg. 2012;256(3):518–28.

Davis S, Raeburn CD. Preoperative laboratory evaluation. In: McIntyre Jr RC, Schulick RD, editors. Surgical decision making. 6th ed. Philadelphia: Elsevier; 2020. p. 2–3.

- Cardiac disease is prevalent among patients undergoing noncardiac surgery. A careful history and physical exam, careful review of electrocardiograms as well as laboratory values afford the clinician the ability to screen for cardiac risk.
- **Risk factors** for cardiac disease include:
  - Age > 55 years.
  - History of prior coronary artery disease (CAD) or myocardial infarction (MI).
  - Prior percutaneous coronary intervention (PCI).
  - Prior coronary artery bypass graft (CABG).
  - History of heart failure.
- Several prediction tools for cardiac risk in noncardiac surgery exist, such as the Revised Cardiac Risk Index, and the NSQIP MI and Cardiac Arrest Calculator. Several patient parameters are used to input and calculate the risk of cardiac events and mortality in patients undergoing surgery.
- Patients with active major cardiac clinical predictors should be stabilized before surgery. These predictors include:
  - STEMI
  - Non-STEMI
  - Unstable angina
  - Decompensated heart failure
  - Arrhythmia
  - Valve disease
- Surgical procedural risk is classified as low risk (<1%) for a major adverse cardiac event (MACE), and elevated risk (>1%) MACE.
- Low-risk MACE procedures include inguinal herniorrhaphy, breast biopsies, and procedures in which low fluid/volume shifts occur. Surgery may proceed without further cardiac evaluation in these cases.
- Elevated risk MACE procedures include major intra-abdominal surgery, intrathoracic procedures, infra-inguinal vascular surgery, and emergency surgery. In these cases, preoperative cardiac evaluation is advised.
- Noninvasive cardiac stress evaluation tests include treadmill + continuous ECG (Bruce protocol), as well as pharmacologically induced cardiac stress + imaging. Dobutamine, adenosine, and dipyridamole are used for stress induction. An echocardiogram or thallium/SESTAMIBI nuclear scan is used for cardiac imaging.
- If significant cardiac lesions are found on these tests, patients must proceed to invasive testing (percutaneous coronary angiography) ± revascularization.
- Regarding perioperative use of β-blockers, these should be continued if they are chronically administered. Starting β-blockers within 24 h of major procedures may reduce the incidence of nonfatal MI. However, there is an increased risk of stroke, bradycardia, hypotension, and death if drug dosing is not titrated to prevent perioperative hypotension.
- Patients with stent placement after PCI are on chronic antiplatelet therapy (frequently dual therapy). When bare metal stents are placed, antiplatelet medications cannot be stopped for 30 days. When drug-eluting stents are placed, antiplatelet medications cannot be stopped for 1 year. Elective noncardiac surgery should be planned accordingly.
- Appropriate timing for antiplatelet/anticoagulant cessation prior to surgery may reduce perioperative bleeding complications. The risk of thrombotic/embolic events secondary to drug cessation should be assessed as well.
  - Clopidogrel/aspirin: hold for 7 days
  - Coumadin can be reversed with vitamin K and FFP
  - Rivaroxaban: hold for 1–3 days
  - Apixaban: hold for 1–3 days
  - Dabitragan: hold for 2–4 days
- Emergency reversal of anticoagulant drugs:
  - Dabitragan: idarucizumab
  - Apixaban/rivaroxaban: andexanet-α, prothrombin complex concentrate (PCC)

C. P. Spanos, *Acute Surgical Topics*, https://doi.org/10.1007/978-3-030-68700-7_2

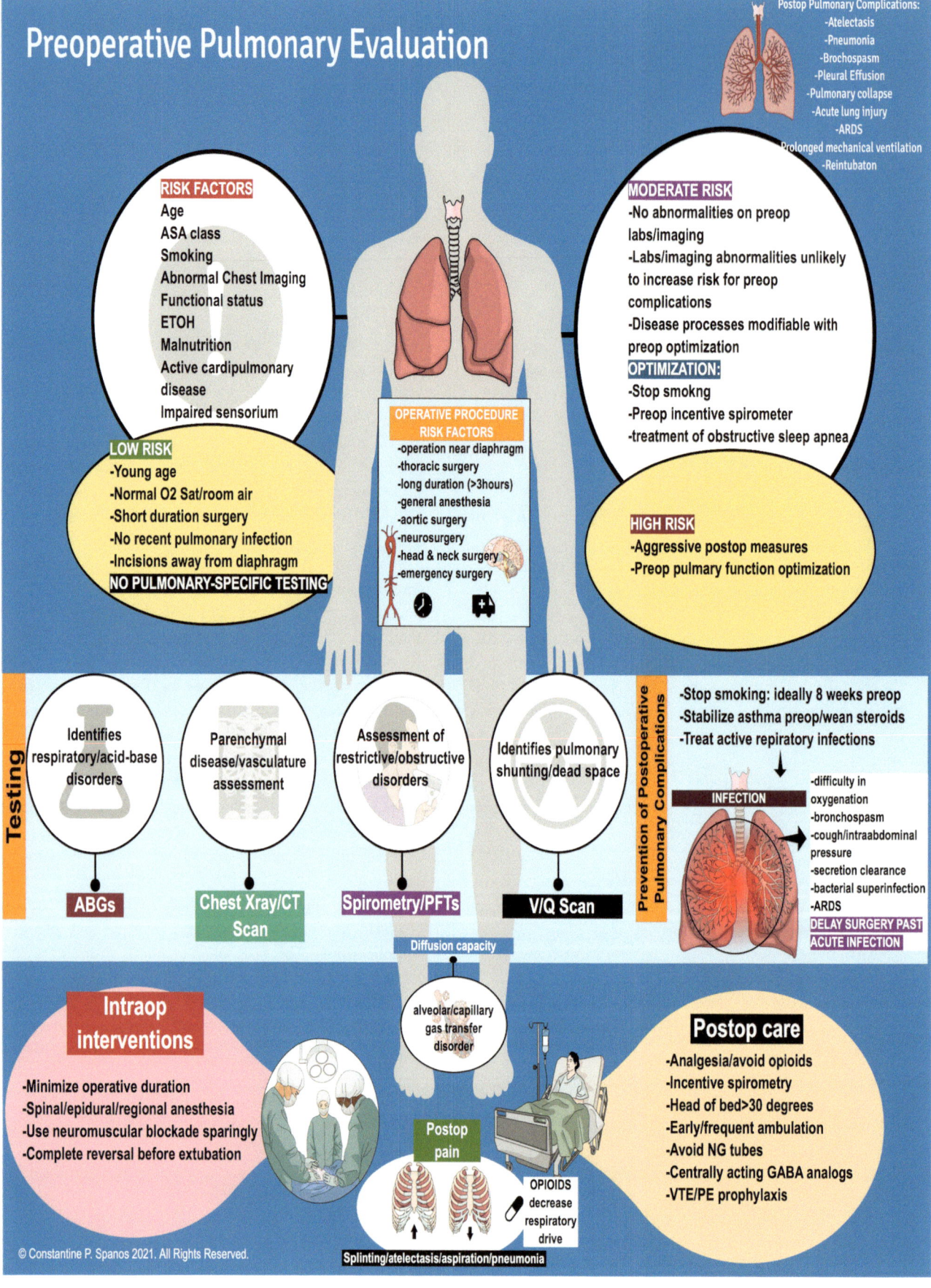

Preoperative Pulmonary Evaluation

Postop Pulmonary Complications:
-Atelectasis
-Pneumonia
-Brochospasm
-Pleural Effusion
-Pulmonary collapse
-Acute lung injury
-ARDS
-Prolonged mechanical ventilation
-Reintubaton

RISK FACTORS
Age
ASA class
Smoking
Abnormal Chest Imaging
Functional status
ETOH
Malnutrition
Active cardipulmonary disease
Impaired sensorium

MODERATE RISK
-No abnormalities on preop labs/imaging
-Labs/imaging abnormalities unlikely to increase risk for preop complications
-Disease processes modifiable with preop optimization
OPTIMIZATION:
-Stop smokng
-Preop incentive spirometer
-treatment of obstructive sleep apnea

LOW RISK
-Young age
-Normal O2 Sat/room air
-Short duration surgery
-No recent pulmonary infection
-Incisions away from diaphragm
NO PULMONARY-SPECIFIC TESTING

OPERATIVE PROCEDURE RISK FACTORS
-operation near diaphragm
-thoracic surgery
-long duration (>3hours)
-general anesthesia
-aortic surgery
-neurosurgery
-head & neck surgery
-emergency surgery

HIGH RISK
-Aggressive postop measures
-Preop pulmary function optimization

Testing

Identifies respiratory/acid-base disorders
ABGs

Parenchymal disease/vasculature assessment
Chest Xray/CT Scan

Assessment of restrictive/obstructive disorders
Spirometry/PFTs

Identifies pulmonary shunting/dead space
V/Q Scan

Prevention of Postoperative Pulmonary Complications
-Stop smoking: ideally 8 weeks preop
-Stabilize asthma preop/wean steroids
-Treat active repiratory infections

INFECTION
-difficulty in oxygenation
-bronchospasm
-cough/intraabdominal pressure
-secretion clearance
-bacterial superinfection
-ARDS
DELAY SURGERY PAST ACUTE INFECTION

Diffusion capacity
alveolar/capillary gas transfer disorder

Intraop interventions
-Minimize operative duration
-Spinal/epidural/regional anesthesia
-Use neuromuscular blockade sparingly
-Complete reversal before extubation

Postop pain
OPIOIDS decrease respiratory drive
Splinting/atelectasis/aspiration/pneumonia

Postop care
-Analgesia/avoid opioids
-Incentive spirometry
-Head of bed>30 degrees
-Early/frequent ambulation
-Avoid NG tubes
-Centrally acting GABA analogs
-VTE/PE prophylaxis

Further Reading

Fleisher LA, Fleischmann KE, Auerbach AD, et al. 2014 ACC/AHA guideline on perioperative cardiovascular evaluation and management of patients undergoing noncardiac surgery: a report of the American College of Cardiology/American Heart Association task force on practice guidelines. J Am Coll Cardiol. 2014;64:e77–e137.

Reece TB, Cleveland JC Jr. Preoperative cardiac evaluation. In: McIntyre Jr RC, Schulick RD, editors. Surgical decision making. 6th ed. Philadelphia: Elsevier; 2020. p. 4–5.

- Pulmonary disease may cause significant morbidity in surgical patients. A careful history and physical exam, careful review of chest X-rays, and laboratory values afford the clinician the ability to screen for pulmonary risk.
- Postoperative pulmonary **complications** include:
  - Atelectasis
  - Pneumonia
  - Bronchospasm
  - Pleural effusion
  - Pulmonary collapse
  - Acute lung injury
  - ARDS
  - Prolonged mechanical ventilation
  - Re-intubation
- **Risk factors** for pulmonary disease include advanced age, ASA class, smoking, abnormal chest X-ray, functional status, alcohol consumption, malnutrition, active cardiopulmonary disease, and impaired sensorium.
- The **type of surgery** also confers risk of postoperative pulmonary complications. Higher risk operations include:
  - Operations near the diaphragm
  - Thoracic surgery
  - Long duration of surgery
  - Aortic surgery
  - Neurosurgery
  - Head and neck surgery
  - Emergency surgery
  - General intubated surgery
- Low-risk parameters for pulmonary complications include:
  - Young patients
  - Normal O_2 saturation on room air
  - Quick surgery
  - Absence of recent pulmonary infection
  - Incisions away from the diaphragm
  In these patients, no pulmonary-specific testing is recommended.

- Moderate-risk patients have disease processes that can be modified preoperatively with smoking cessation, pulmonary physiotherapy with an incentive spirometer, and treatment of obstructive sleep apnea.
- High-risk patients need preoperative pulmonary function optimization and aggressive postoperative pulmonary management, discussed below.
- Tests and imaging can assess pulmonary lesions quantitatively and qualitatively.
- An arterial blood gas (ABG) may identify respiratory and acid-base disorders.
- A chest X-ray or a CT scan may identify parenchymal disease and assess pulmonary vasculature.
- Spirometry and pulmonary function tests (PFTs) are used to assess restrictive and obstructive pulmonary disorders.
- Diffusion capacity can be used to identify alveolar/capillary gas transfer disorders.
- Ventilation/perfusion scans identify pulmonary shunting and dead space.
- Prevention of postoperative pulmonary complications can be achieved by:
  - Smoking cessation 8 weeks prior to surgery.
  - Stabilization of asthma/steroid wean.
  - Treatment of active pulmonary infections. Surgery should be delayed past active infection. Infection can cause oxygenation impairment, bronchospasm, increased coughing/intra-abdominal pressure, impair secretion clearance, cause superinfection and ARDS.
- Intraoperative interventions that may reduce pulmonary complications include minimization of surgical time, the use of spinal, epidural or regional anesthesia, sparse use of neuromuscular blockade, and complete anesthetic reversal before extubation.
- Postoperatively, pulmonary complications can be mitigated by optimal pain control, avoiding opioids, early ambulation, elevation of the head of the bed to avoid aspiration, avoiding nasogastric tubes, and VTE prophylaxis.

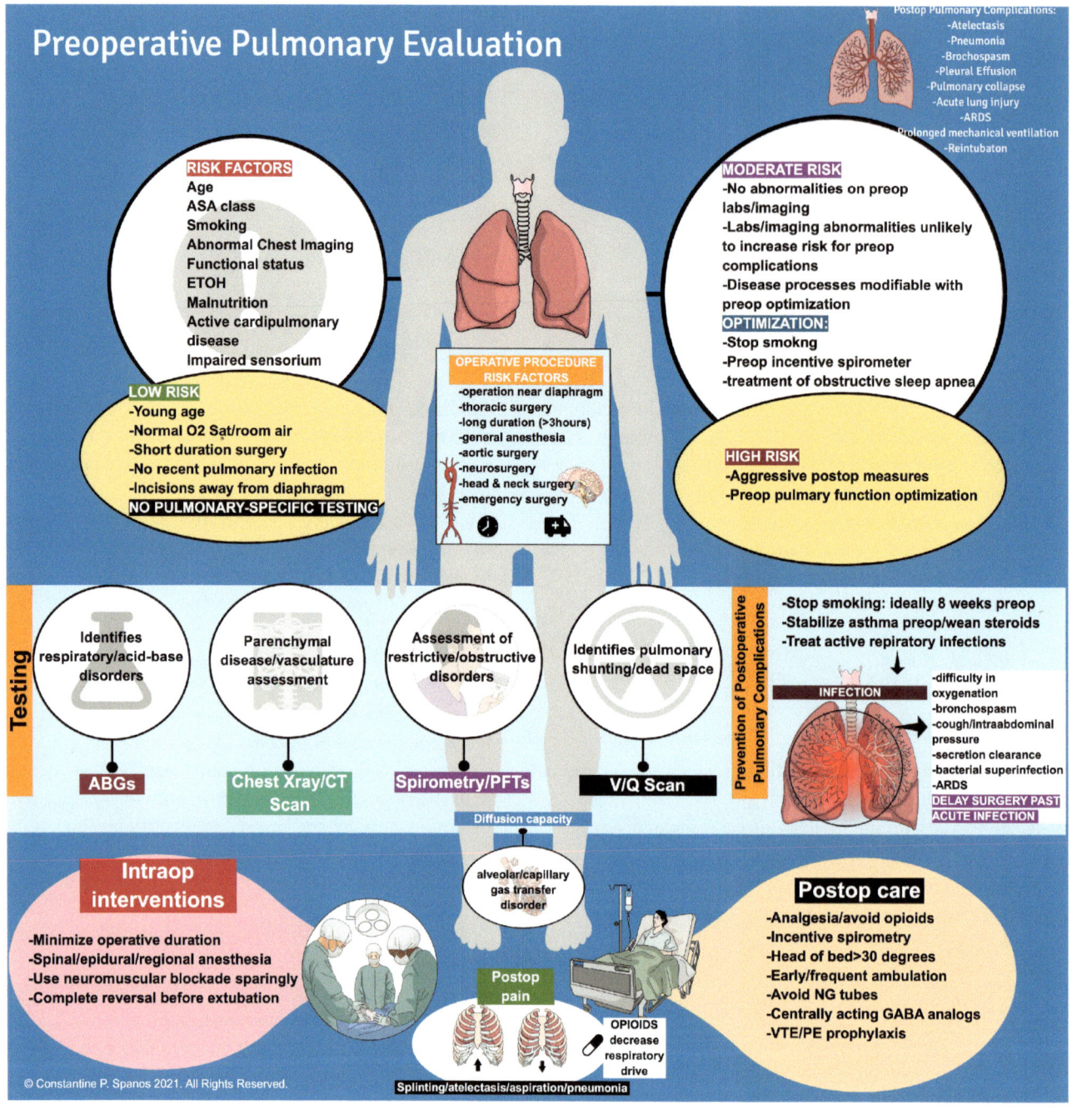

Preoperative Pulmonary Evaluation

Postop Pulmonary Complications:
- Atelectasis
- Pneumonia
- Brochospasm
- Pleural Effusion
- Pulmonary collapse
- Acute lung injury
- ARDS
- Prolonged mechanical ventilation
- Reintubaton

RISK FACTORS
Age
ASA class
Smoking
Abnormal Chest Imaging
Functional status
ETOH
Malnutrition
Active cardipulmonary disease
Impaired sensorium

MODERATE RISK
-No abnormalities on preop labs/imaging
-Labs/imaging abnormalities unlikely to increase risk for preop complications
-Disease processes modifiable with preop optimization
OPTIMIZATION:
-Stop smokng
-Preop incentive spirometer
-treatment of obstructive sleep apnea

LOW RISK
-Young age
-Normal O2 Sat/room air
-Short duration surgery
-No recent pulmonary infection
-Incisions away from diaphragm
NO PULMONARY-SPECIFIC TESTING

OPERATIVE PROCEDURE RISK FACTORS
-operation near diaphragm
-thoracic surgery
-long duration (>3hours)
-general anesthesia
-aortic surgery
-neurosurgery
-head & neck surgery
-emergency surgery

HIGH RISK
-Aggressive postop measures
-Preop pulmary function optimization

Testing

Identifies respiratory/acid-base disorders
ABGs

Parenchymal disease/vasculature assessment
Chest Xray/CT Scan

Assessment of restrictive/obstructive disorders
Spirometry/PFTs

Identifies pulmonary shunting/dead space
V/Q Scan

Prevention of Postoperative Pulmonary Complications
-Stop smoking: ideally 8 weeks preop
-Stabilize asthma preop/wean steroids
-Treat active repiratory infections

INFECTION
-difficulty in oxygenation
-bronchospasm
-cough/intraabdominal pressure
-secretion clearance
-bacterial superinfection
-ARDS
DELAY SURGERY PAST ACUTE INFECTION

Diffusion capacity

alveolar/capillary gas transfer disorder

Intraop interventions

-Minimize operative duration
-Spinal/epidural/regional anesthesia
-Use neuromuscular blockade sparingly
-Complete reversal before extubation

Postop pain

OPIOIDS decrease respiratory drive

Splinting/atelectasis/aspiration/pneumonia

Postop care

-Analgesia/avoid opioids
-Incentive spirometry
-Head of bed>30 degrees
-Early/frequent ambulation
-Avoid NG tubes
-Centrally acting GABA analogs
-VTE/PE prophylaxis

Further Reading

Brooks-Brunn JA. Predictors of postoperative pulmonary complications following abdominal surgery. Chest. 1997;111(3):564.

Hoffmann JRH, Meguid RA. Preoperative pulmonary evaluation. In: McIntyre Jr RC, Schulick RD, editors. Surgical decision making. 6th ed. Philadelphia: Elsevier; 2020. p. 6–7.

- Medical imaging can be extremely useful when encountering acute surgical problems. It is an important adjunct in making a diagnosis, and may guide treatment.
- Not all patients with acute surgical conditions need imaging. A careful history and physical exam will often lead to a correct clinical diagnosis. Medical imaging may narrow down an extensive differential diagnosis, classify a diagnosis that has already been made (i.e., acute pancreatitis), and facilitate operative planning.
- The ABCs of medical imaging provide a simple method of reviewing images by a non-radiologist clinician, facilitating diagnostic skills. It is mostly useful with plain films and CT scans. Reading ultrasonic images requires more of a learning curve, and MRI scans are a little more complex than CT scans.
- Ideally, images are reviewed with a radiologist; clinical correlation with the physician providing care (surgeon, internist, etc.) increases diagnostic accuracy and may prove educational for everyone involved. **Merely waiting for a radiological report on an ordered test is unacceptable**.
- The ABCs are based on the fact that most images depict different tissue densities. In most plain films and CT scans, air is black, and all other tissue, fluid, contrast, and calcifications are of higher density.
- **A = Air**. In most medical images, air is **normally** found in the following:
  - Trachea
  - Bronchi
  - Alveoli
  - Stomach (gastric bubble)
  - Small intestine
  - Colon
  - Rectum
- Air in the following regions is considered **abnormal**:
  - Subcutaneous tissue (subcutaneous emphysema)
  - Pleural space (pneumothorax)
  - Peritoneal cavity (free intraperitoneal air/ pneumoperitoneum)
  - Bowel wall (pneumatosis intestinalis)
  - Biliary tree
  - Portal venous circulation
  - Solid organ parenchyma
- Normal and abnormal **air patterns** should also be noted. Examples are air-fluid levels (small bowel obstruction), a large gastric bubble, and colonic distention.
- **B = Bone**. Significant findings regarding bony structures include:
  - Fracture
  - Displacement
  - Joint abnormalities
  - Asymmetry
  - Anatomic/congenital abnormality
  - Developmental abnormalities
  - Osteoporosis/osteopenia
  - Hardware (orthopedic interventions, prostheses)
- **C = Content, calcification, contrast**.
- Look at the corresponding **anatomical content** in the medical image (i.e., cardiac silhouette, bowel, airway):
  - Is the morphology normal?
  - Is the size normal?
  - Is there symmetry?
  - Is the content displaced?
  - Is there missing anatomy? Is other hardware present (pacemaker + wires, central venous lines, chemotherapy port)?
  - Also, check for A, B in this area.
- **Calcifications** are associated with and may depict:
  - Aortic aneurysms
    Peripheral vascular disease
  - Phleboliths
  - Urinary stones
  - Gallstones
  - Thyroid nodules (ultrasound)
  - Breast disorders
- **Radiopaque contrast** is frequently used in medical imaging. It may be administered intravascularly, via the gastrointestinal tract or the urinary tract. Significant findings after use of contrast in imaging include:

© The Author(s), under exclusive license to Springer Nature Switzerland AG 2021
C. P. Spanos, *Acute Surgical Topics*, https://doi.org/10.1007/978-3-030-68700-7_4

- Extravasation (bleeding, anastomotic leak)
- Luminal stenosis (bowel obstruction)
- Filling defects (common bile duct stones)
- Dilation
- Reflux
- Abnormal communication (fistula)
- **D = density, distention, dilation**. Careful observation of normal/abnormal densities in a medical image may lead to diagnosis of a mass, infiltrations on a chest X-ray, pleural effusion, and hemothorax. In a CT scan, a reference to the Hounsfield density scale is useful.
- **E = extravasation**, extra-anatomical location (i.e., stomach in the chest in a paraesophageal hernia).

The ABC's of Medical Imaging

Imaging is an important adjunct in making a diagnosis. One must use sound judgement regarding both the necessity as well as the type of imaging to be performed. Careful use of these basic ABC's may help most clinicians detect abnormalities in most images. Merely waiting for a radiological report on your patient is not acceptable.

A=Air

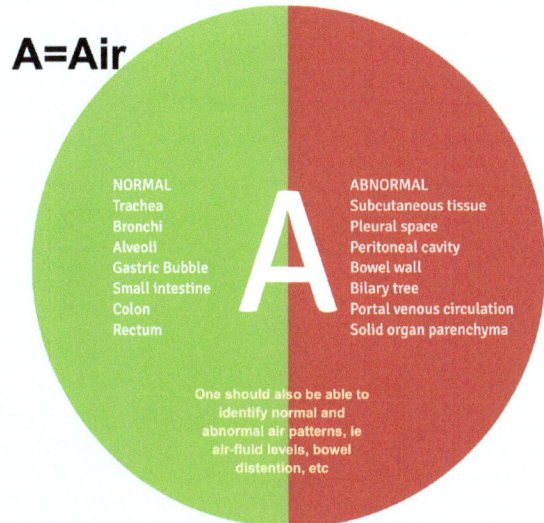

NORMAL
Trachea
Bronchi
Alveoli
Gastric Bubble
Small intestine
Colon
Rectum

ABNORMAL
Subcutaneous tissue
Pleural space
Peritoneal cavity
Bowel wall
Bilary tree
Portal venous circulation
Solid organ parenchyma

One should also be able to identify normal and abnormal air patterns, ie air-fluid levels, bowel distention, etc

B=Bone

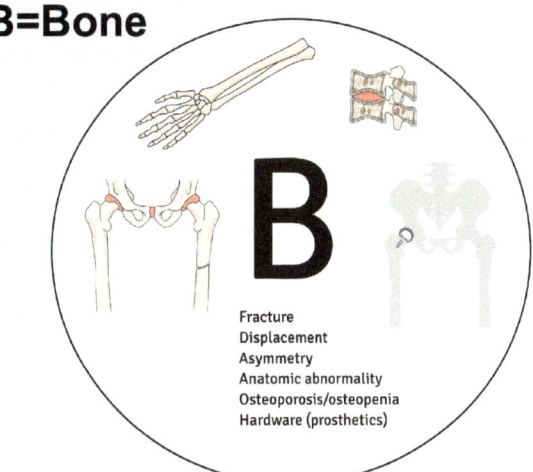

Fracture
Displacement
Asymmetry
Anatomic abnormality
Osteoporosis/osteopenia
Hardware (prosthetics)

C=Content, Calcification, Contrast

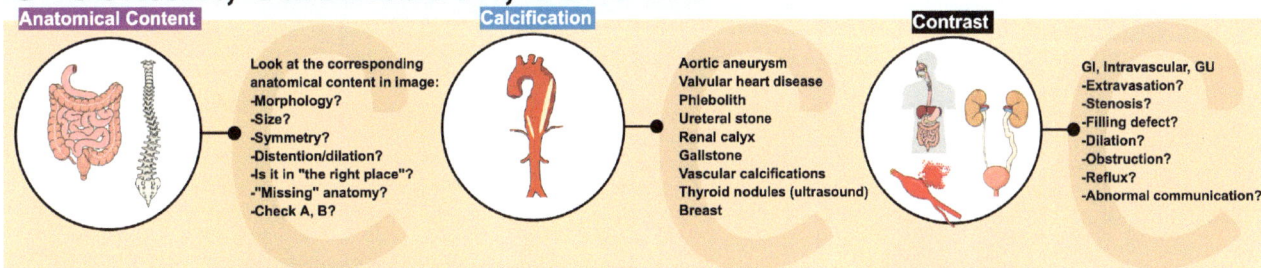

Anatomical Content

Look at the corresponding anatomical content in image:
-Morphology?
-Size?
-Symmetry?
-Distention/dilation?
-Is it in "the right place"?
-"Missing" anatomy?
-Check A, B?

Calcification

Aortic aneurysm
Valvular heart disease
Phlebolith
Ureteral stone
Renal calyx
Gallstone
Vascular calcifications
Thyroid nodules (ultrasound)
Breast

Contrast

GI, Intravascular, GU
-Extravasation?
-Stenosis?
-Filling defect?
-Dilation?
-Obstruction?
-Reflux?
-Abnormal communication?

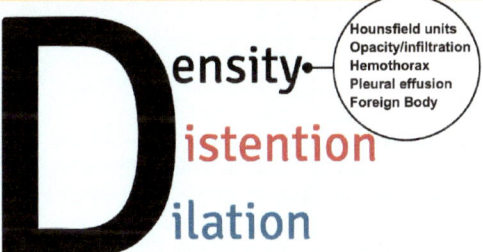

Density
Distention
Dilation

Hounsfield units
Opacity/infiltration
Hemothorax
Pleural effusion
Foreign Body

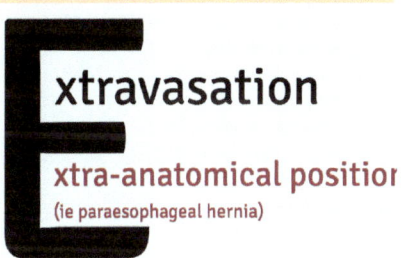

Extravasation
Extra-anatomical position
(ie paraesophageal hernia)

Further Reading

Silen W. Laboratory and radiological tests. In: Silen W, editor. Cope's early diagnosis of the acute abdomen. 22nd ed. New York: Oxford University Press; 2010. p. 54–66.

- Acute appendicitis is the most common acute abdominal disorder encountered in daily practice. It occurs in 7–12% of the population; peak incidence is in the second to third decade of life. Surgeons are consulted most frequently to either diagnose or "rule out" acute appendicitis by their colleagues in general medicine or pediatrics. Early diagnosis leads to timely and frequently uncomplicated treatment of this disorder; conversely, delay in diagnosis may increase morbidity of both the disorder and operative treatment. A thorough understanding of the etiopathogenesis, signs and symptoms, physical exam, and adjunctive diagnostic tests and imaging helps greatly in making a timely and accurate diagnosis of appendicitis.

- The most prevalent theory regarding etiology is appendiceal luminal obstruction. This may be mechanical (fecalith, appendicolith), a result of lymphoid hyperplasia or caused by parasites or a neoplasm. Continued mucosal secretion leads to distention and an increase in intraluminal pressure. This, in turn, causes venous outflow obstruction and arterial inflow obstruction. Ischemia leads to inflammation, which progresses from mucosa to serosa. Perforation is the end-result of this process if left untreated.

- The sequence of clinical signs and symptoms reflect the above-mentioned processes. Initially, the patient complains of progressive mid-epigastric discomfort (appendiceal obstruction/distention). This is classical visceral pain. Then anorexia may set in; nausea and vomiting are frequent. Low-grade fever may appear at this point. (Increased appendiceal distention, venous congestion, and increase in peristalsis). After a period of a few hours, the pain localizes in the right lower quadrant; tenderness is elicited by palpation. (Transmural inflammation abutting the overlying parietal peritoneum). This is classic somatic pain. Constitutional signs such as fever and mild tachycardia may appear at this point. Perforation results in intense localized pain, diffuse abdominal pain, and high fever.

- **Vomiting after pain** is common in acute appendicitis; vomiting **before** the onset of pain should lead to other diagnostic considerations.

- The classic appendicitis sequence may not be present in all cases; patients may underestimate the initial symptoms and not report them; patients at the extremes of ages and those on chronic analgesic or immunosuppressant medications may have attenuation of signs and symptoms.

- Acute appendicitis can be pathologically classified as follows:
  - **Mucosal**; occurs usually less than 24 h in the process. Nonoperative therapy is most successful with this type.
  - **Phlegmonous**; occurs within 24 h and is characterized by transmural inflammation. Nonoperative therapy is not as successful.
  - **Necrotic**; usually associated with contained or free perforation. This may lead to generalized peritonitis, phlegmon, and/or abscess.

- The most common flora associated with appendicitis are Gram-negative aerobic and anaerobic enteric flora; this may guide antibiotic prophylaxis prior to surgery, antibiotic treatment in perforated appendicitis, and nonoperative treatment of appendicitis.

- Patients in the early stages of appendicitis appear slightly unwell. Palpation in the RLQ elicits tenderness (**McBurney's sign**); palpation in the LLQ elicits pain in the RLQ (**Rovsing's sign**). Hyperextension of the flexed right extremity when in the left lateral decubitus position elicits right-sided pain (**iliopsoas sign**). Medial and lateral rotation of the thigh elicits hypogastric pain (**obturator sign**). Patients in later stages of appendicitis appear quite unwell.

- Perforation is frequently the result of delay in diagnosis and treatment. Morbidity (and mortality!) increases and operative treatment becomes complex. Free perforation leads to generalized peritonitis; contained perforation may lead to a phlegmon and/or abscess. Primary operative treatment of the latter two conditions results in extensive, morbid operations and is usually not recommended.

- Diagnostic testing includes laboratory tests and imaging.
- The most common labs used to aid in the diagnosis of acute appendicitis are the complete blood count (CBC) and C-reactive protein (CRP). Leukocytosis is common, as is an increased CRP value. A normal WBC **and** CRP are rare in acute appendicitis.
- Imaging modalities used most frequently are plain abdominal films, ultrasound, and computed tomography.
- Acute appendicitis has an extensive medical, surgical, and gynecological differential diagnosis.
  - **Medical:**
    Influenza
    Diaphragmatic pleurisy
    Herpes Zoster infection
    Typhoid fever
    Porphyria
    Gastroenteritis
    Hepatitis
    Diabetic ketoacidosis
    Mesenteric adenitis
  - **Surgical**
    Nephrolithiasis
    Cholecystitis
    Colonic Diverticulitis
    Meckel's diverticulitis
    Omental torsion
    Crohn's disease
    Testicular torsion
  - **Gynecological**
    Mittelschmerz
    Dysmenorrhea
    Acute salpingitis
    Ectopic pregnancy
    Threatened abortion
    Ovarian cyst rupture/torsion

- **Never forget a pregnancy test in females of reproductive age, as well as scrotal palpation in males.**
- Treatment of acute appendicitis is operative and nonoperative. Most cases of appendicitis are treated with open or laparoscopic appendectomy. Generalized peritonitis mandates operation. An appendiceal phlegmon is usually treated with antibiotic therapy, followed by interval appendectomy at 3 months. Appendiceal abscesses are usually drained by interventional radiology, followed by interval appendectomy at 3 months. Nonoperative treatment of appendicitis is acceptable in cases of early, mucosal, clinically mild disease. There is a risk of early or late recurrence.
- **Nonoperative treatment of appendicitis always runs the risk of missing the rare appendiceal neoplasm (adenocarcinoma, carcinoid).**
- **Always remember, there are two ways of making the diagnosis of acute appendicitis: either you make the diagnosis or someone makes it for you!**

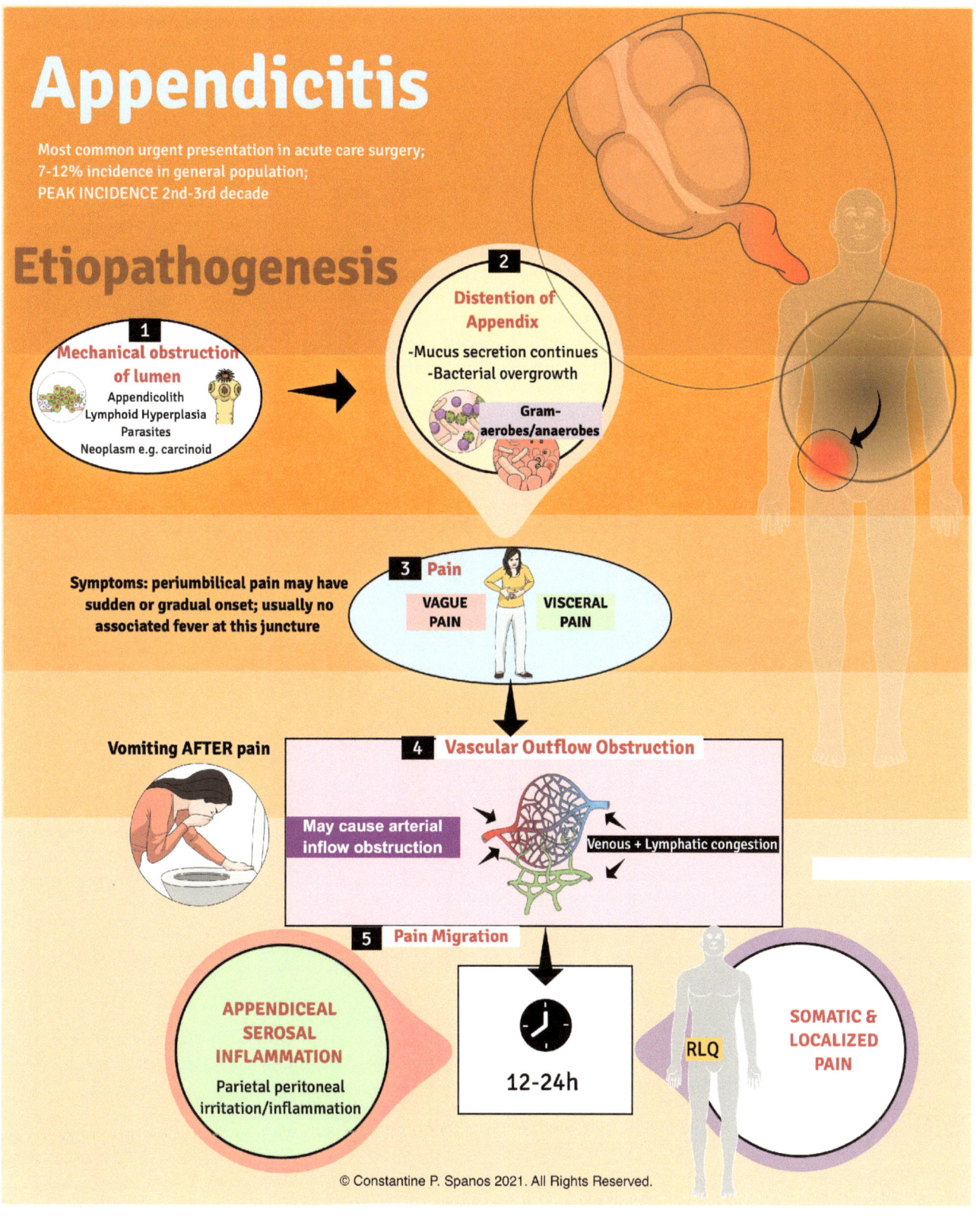

Appendicitis

Most common urgent presentation in acute care surgery;
7-12% incidence in general population;
PEAK INCIDENCE 2nd-3rd decade

Etiopathogenesis

1 Mechanical obstruction of lumen
Appendicolith
Lymphoid Hyperplasia
Parasites
Neoplasm e.g. carcinoid

2 Distention of Appendix
-Mucus secretion continues
-Bacterial overgrowth
Gram- aerobes/anaerobes

Symptoms: periumbilical pain may have sudden or gradual onset; usually no associated fever at this juncture

3 Pain
VAGUE PAIN
VISCERAL PAIN

Vomiting AFTER pain

4 Vascular Outflow Obstruction
May cause arterial inflow obstruction
Venous + Lymphatic congestion

5 Pain Migration

APPENDICEAL SEROSAL INFLAMMATION
Parietal peritoneal irritation/inflammation

12-24h

RLQ

SOMATIC & LOCALIZED PAIN

Appendicitis:
Order of Symptoms

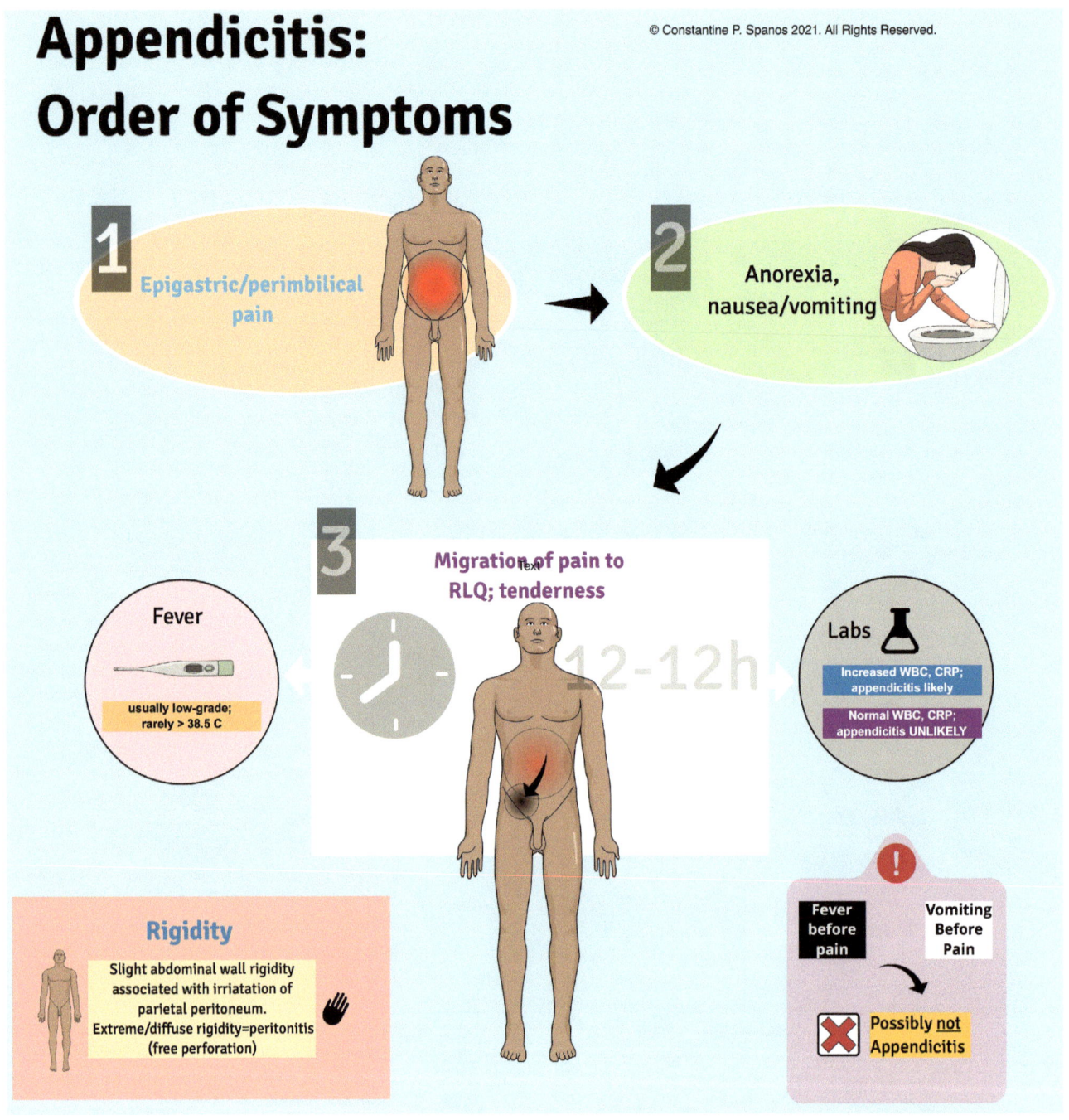

1 Epigastric/perimbilical pain

2 Anorexia, nausea/vomiting

3 Migration of pain to RLQ; tenderness

12-12h

Fever
usually low-grade; rarely > 38.5 C

Labs
Increased WBC, CRP; appendicitis likely
Normal WBC, CRP; appendicitis UNLIKELY

Rigidity
Slight abdominal wall rigidity associated with irriation of parietal peritoneum. Extreme/diffuse rigidity=peritonitis (free perforation)

Fever before pain   Vomiting Before Pain
Possibly *not* Appendicitis

Appendicitis
types:
(pathology/morphology)

from Sir Zachary Cope

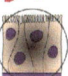

	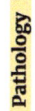Pathology	**Mucosal** Early stage < 24 h	**Phlegmonous** Transmural inflammation Within 24 h	**Necrotic** >24 h Usually associated with perforation
 	Clinical findings Labs / Treatment	Vague pain; tenderness may be non-significant/absent; fever, leukocytosis may be absent; non operative therapy most successful with this type	Pain; RLQ tenderness; fever leukocytosis; non-operative therapy not as successful	Symptoms/signs may be exacerbated; increased morbity of disease and/or surgical treatment; non-operative treatment only if progression to phlegmon/abscess

Microbes

Appendicitis

Gram Negative Aerobes & Anaerobes
E.Coli, B Fragilis, Klebsiella Pneumonia, Streptococcus, Enterococcus, P. Aeruginosa

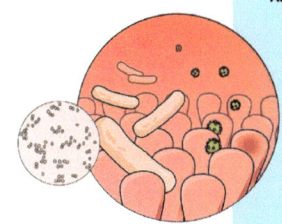

Antibiotic Prophylaxis & Treatment

Knowledge of the usual flora involved in appendicitis is useful:
-Prophylaxis prior to surgery
-Antibiotic treatment in perforated appendicitis (postoperative)
-Non-surgical treatment of appendicitis

Prophylaxis:
Single-dose or 24h of broad-spectrum antibiotic

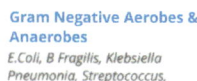

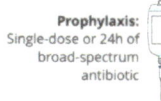

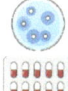

Treatment: empiric broad-spectrum antibiotics; may narrow spectrum based on culture. Duration: 10-14 d empirically, or when signs, symptoms and labs normalize.

Physical Exam

Signs

In appendicitis, we find some notable eponymous physical signs and anatomic points.

Despite the availability of diagnostic imaging, the signs and symptoms, along with a careful history, frequently leads to the diagnosis.

McBurney's Point

RLQ tenderness; Involved parietal peritoneum overlying inflamed appendix

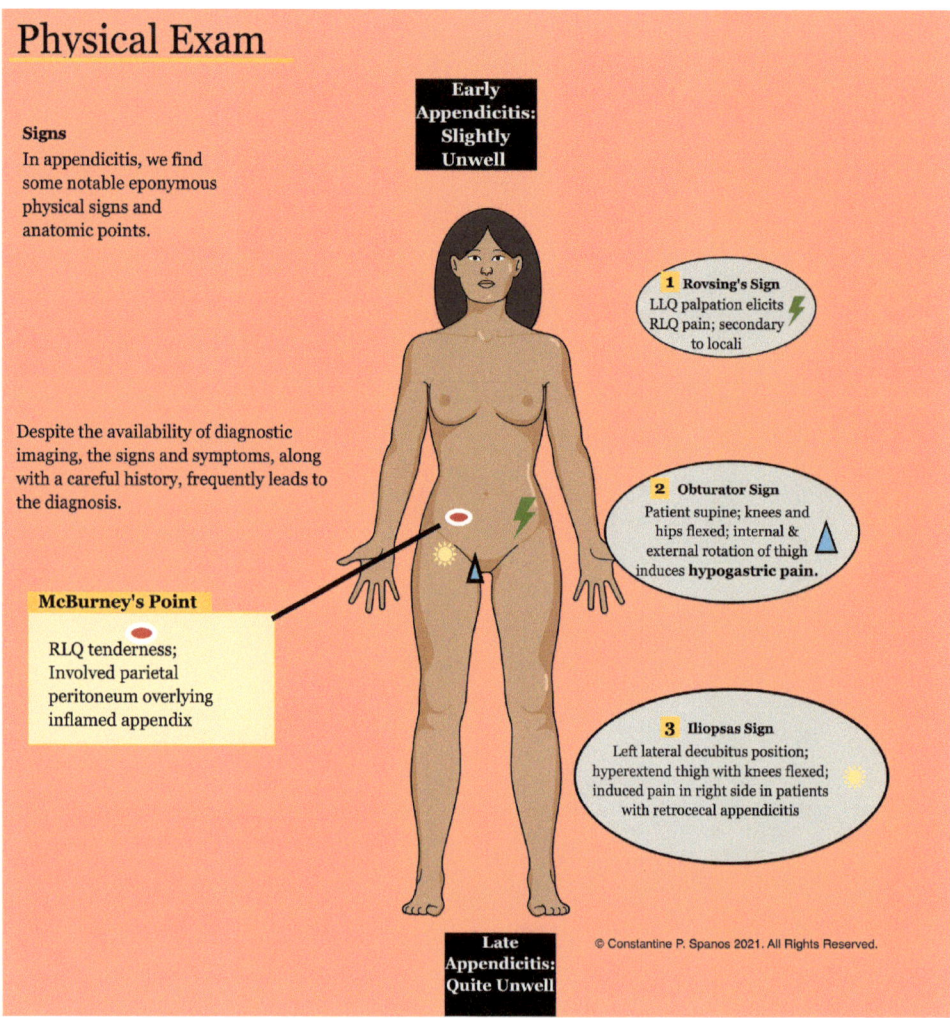

Early Appendicitis: Slightly Unwell

1 Rovsing's Sign
LLQ palpation elicits RLQ pain; secondary to locali

2 Obturator Sign
Patient supine; knees and hips flexed; internal & external rotation of thigh induces **hypogastric pain.**

3 Iliopsas Sign
Left lateral decubitus position; hyperextend thigh with knees flexed; induced pain in right side in patients with retrocecal appendicitis

Late Appendicitis: Quite Unwell

Perforation

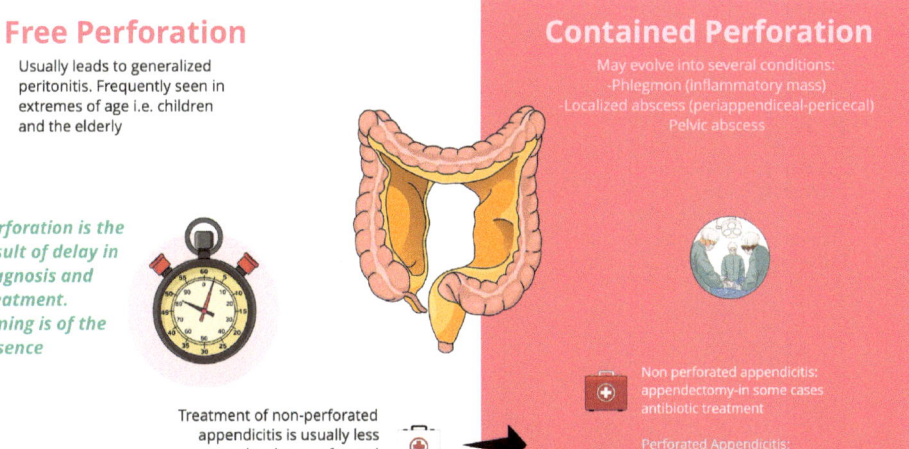

Free Perforation

Usually leads to generalized peritonitis. Frequently seen in extremes of age i.e. children and the elderly

Perforation is the result of delay in diagnosis and treatment. Timing is of the essence

Treatment of non-perforated appendicitis is usually less complex than perforated appendicitis

Contained Perforation

May evolve into several conditions:
-Phlegmon (Inflammatory mass)
-Localized abscess (periappendiceal-pericecal)
Pelvic abscess

Non perforated appendicitis: appendectomy-in some cases antibiotic treatment

Perforated Appendicitis: prolonged antibiotic treatment; percutaneous drainage of abscess; complicated surgery; multiple interventions

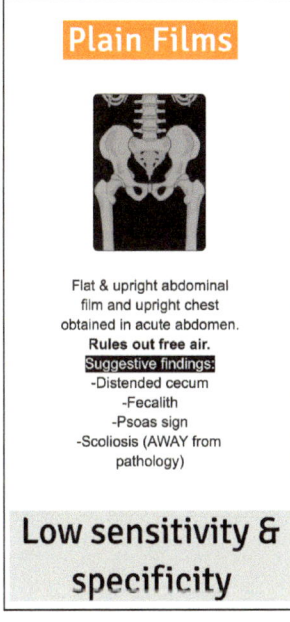

Plain Films

Flat & upright abdominal film and upright chest obtained in acute abdomen.
Rules out free air.
Suggestive findings:
-Distended cecum
-Fecalith
-Psoas sign
-Scoliosis (AWAY from pathology)

Low sensitivity & specificity

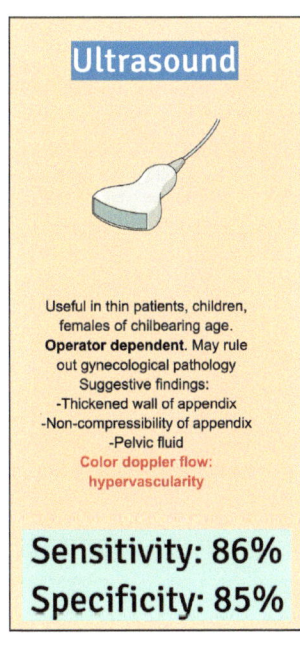

Ultrasound

Useful in thin patients, children, females of chilbearing age.
Operator dependent. May rule out gynecological pathology
Suggestive findings:
-Thickened wall of appendix
-Non-compressibility of appendix
-Pelvic fluid
Color doppler flow: hypervascularity

Sensitivity: 86%
Specificity: 85%

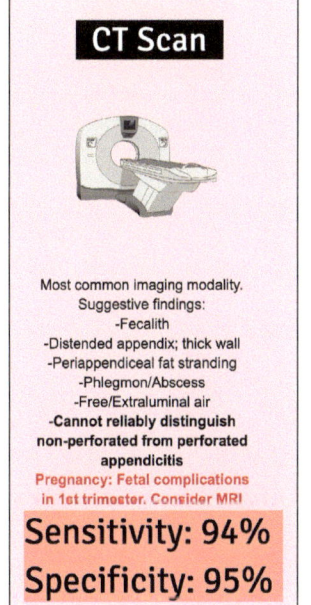

CT Scan

Most common imaging modality.
Suggestive findings:
-Fecalith
-Distended appendix; thick wall
-Periappendiceal fat stranding
-Phlegmon/Abscess
-Free/Extraluminal air
-Cannot reliably distinguish non-perforated from perforated appendicitis
Pregnancy: Fetal complications in 1st trimester. Consider MRI

Sensitivity: 94%
Specificity: 95%

"There are two ways to make the diagnosis of appendicitis...either you make the diagnosis, or someone makes the diagnosis for you..."

-C. Spanos, MD

Appendicitis: Differential Diagnosis I

Appendicitis has a notoriously extensive
differential diagnosis. Here's where the
clinician in you will shine.

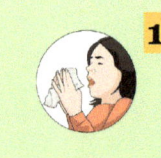

1 Influenza
Abdominal pain usually
more generalized; back
pain; headache; upper
respiratory symptoms;
vomiting BEFORE pain

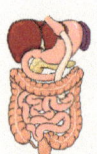 **6 Gastroenteritis**

Diffuse abdominal pain;
cramping; intense
nausea/vomiting±diarrhea.
Tenderness/rigidity usually
absent

 **2 Diaphragmatic
Pleurisy**

Early basal pneumonia; deep
palpation in RLQ <u>does not</u>
increase pain; Rovsing sign
absent; RR increased, no
abdominal wall rigidity.
Auscultation, CXR aids in
diagnosis

5 Porphyria

 Porphyrinogen precursor accumulation; abdominal
pain attacks; porphyria cutanea tarda reddish-brown
urine; peripheral neuropathy, seizures; psychosis.
Induced by drugs: EtOH, diclofenac, contraceptives,
TCA, benzodiazepines, anesthetics, abx.
Porphobilinogen in urine; coproporphyrin III in
urine/stool

 3 Herpes Zoster

May cause pain
referred to the
appendicular region;
prodromic pain prior to
appearance of
cutaneous lesions

4 Typhoid/Enteric Fever

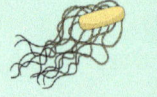 RLQ tenderness; headache;
high fever; general malaise;
profound diarrhea; roseola;
splenomegaly; +agglutination
reaction

Appendicitis: Differential Diagnosis II

		you may be tricked by:	But...
Hepatitis		Abdominal pain; nausea; vomiting; anorexia	Usually no RLQ localization; +jaundice; abnormal LFT's
Diabetic Ketoacidosis		severe abdominal pain; abdominal wall rigidity	History of diabetes; hyperglycemia; ketones in urine; abdominal lesions may precipitate ketoacidosis
Cholecystitits		pain, vomiting; fever; local right-sided tenderness	Pain usually higher; pain in right subscapular region, Murphy's (deep tenderness in right hypochondrium
Nephrolithiasis Pyonephrosis Perinephric abscess		abdominal pain; may localize in RLQ; nausea and vomiting	Pyuria; constitutional symptoms; toxemia; may not have initial epigastric pain/rigidity; anterior abdominal tenderness absent; tenderness in erector-costal angle below last rib; in 80%: stone visible on plain radiograph; testicular pain.

Appendicitis: Differential Diagnosis III

		Clinical characteristics	But:
Crohn's disease		RLQ pain; tenderness; nausea/vomiting	May have history of previous attacks; palpable mass leans towards Crohn's diagnosis; imaging
Omental Torsion		RLQ pain and tenderness	Vomiting less common; initial mid-epigastric pain usually absent; imaging
Diverticulitis		Right-sided diverticulitis and redundant sigmoid anatomy may have similar clinical findings to appendicitis	Initial mid-epigastric pain absent; nausea/vomiting uncommon; fever usually higher; imaging
Meckel's Diverticulitis		May be indistinguishable from appendicitis clinically	Pain may be central and poorly localized; rare (2% of population)
Mesenteric Adenitis		RLQ tenderness, colicky abdominal pain	Nausea/vomiting usually absent; no progression; recent history of viral infection; *Yersinia Enterocollica* common cause

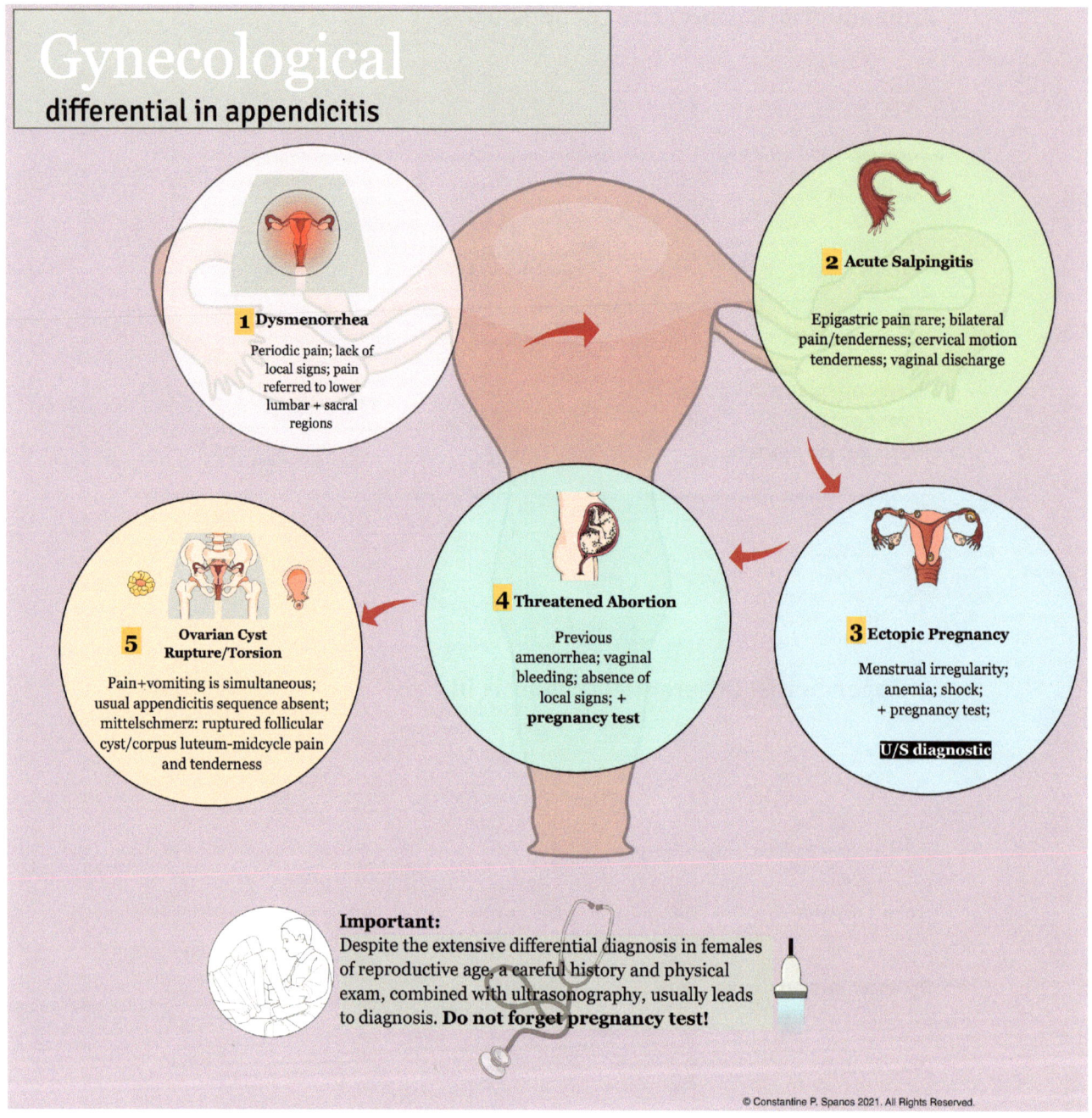

Gynecological
differential in appendicitis

1 Dysmenorrhea

Periodic pain; lack of local signs; pain referred to lower lumbar + sacral regions

2 Acute Salpingitis

Epigastric pain rare; bilateral pain/tenderness; cervical motion tenderness; vaginal discharge

3 Ectopic Pregnancy

Menstrual irregularity; anemia; shock; + pregnancy test;

U/S diagnostic

4 Threatened Abortion

Previous amenorrhea; vaginal bleeding; absence of local signs; + **pregnancy test**

5 Ovarian Cyst Rupture/Torsion

Pain+vomiting is simultaneous; usual appendicitis sequence absent; mittelschmerz: ruptured follicular cyst/corpus luteum-midcycle pain and tenderness

Important:
Despite the extensive differential diagnosis in females of reproductive age, a careful history and physical exam, combined with ultrasonography, usually leads to diagnosis. **Do not forget pregnancy test!**

Appendicitis: Treatment

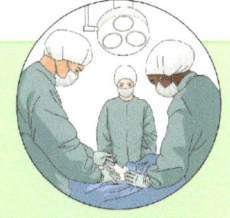

Operative Treatment

Ideally, within 24h. Open or laparoscopic appendectomy. Benefits of laparoscopy include fewer wound infections, shorter length of stay, quicker return to activities. Also better for diagnostic uncertainty, increased BMI

Perforated-generalized peritonitis: operative therapy mandatory

 Surgery after an in-hopsital delay of 12h vs 24h not associated with increased risk of perforation

Delay of >48h increases the risk of surgical site infections and other complications

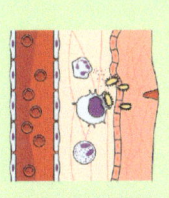 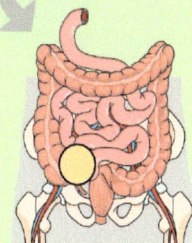

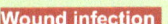

Wound infection   **Abscess**

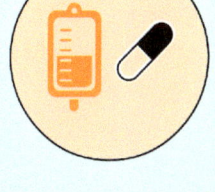

Non-operative Treatment

Non-perforated: empiric broad-spectrum IV antibiotics;
serial examination; possible serial imaging.
10% failure rate on initial admission

Phlegmon: Empiric broad-spectrum IV antibiotics; interval appendectomy after 6-12 weeks

Abscess: Image-guided drainage + antibiotics; interval appendectomy after 6-12 weeks

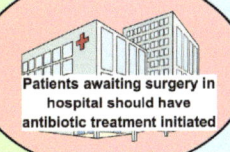
Patients awaiting surgery in hospital should have antibiotic treatment initiated

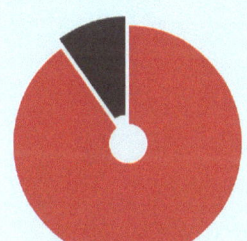

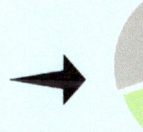

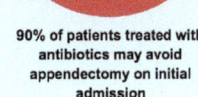

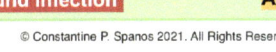

90% of patients treated with antibiotics may avoid appendectomy on initial admission

70% of patients treated with antibiotics may avoid appendectomy the first year; 30% will require surgery (mean time 4-7 months)

Further Reading

Acute appendicitis. In: McLatchie G, Borley N, Chikwe J, editors. Oxford handbook of clinical surgery. 4th ed. Oxford: Oxford University Press; 2013. p. 298–9.

Chung H, Bochicchio G. The acute abdomen. In: Klingensmith ME, Vemuri C, Fayanju OM, Robertson JO, Samson JO, Sanford D, editors. The Washington manual of surgery. 7th ed. Philadelphia: Wolters Kluwer; 2016. p. 279–98.

Shakoor A, Pegoli W Jr. The management of acute appendicitis. In: Cameron JL, Cameron AM, editors. Current surgical therapy. 12th ed. Philadelphia: Elsevier; 2017. p. 265–70.

Silen W. Appendicitis. In: Silen W, editor. Cope's early diagnosis of the acute abdomen. 22nd ed. New York: Oxford University Press; 2010. p. 67–104.

- Cholecystopathy, namely, disorders of the gallbladder, is caused by gallstones in the majority of cases. The cholecystopathies are an assortment of disorders, each of which has characteristic signs and symptoms.
- The incidence of gallstones (cholelithiasis) in the general population is 10–15%. Cholecystopathy will develop in approximately 20% of individuals with gallstones. Advanced age, female sex, and obesity are risk factors for gallstone development.
- The three main types of gallstones are cholesterol, pigment, and mixed stones. Each type has morphologic characteristics and is associated with specific risk factors and epidemiologic groups.
- The most common cholecystopathies are:
  – Symptomatic cholelithiasis
  – Biliary colic
  – Acute cholecystitis
  – Choledocholithiasis/cholangitis
  – Gallstone pancreatitis
  – Gallstone ileus
- **Symptomatic cholelithiasis** is characterized by vague epigastric/RUQ pain following a meal. Pain is usually of low intensity; radiation to the right scapula is frequent. There may be associated nausea and vomiting. Tenderness and fever are absent, and labs are for the most part normal. Diagnosis is confirmed by abdominal ultrasound. Elective laparoscopic cholecystectomy is the treatment of choice.
- **Biliary colic** is caused by temporary impaction of a gallstone in the cystic duct. Symptoms develop rapidly; there is an onset of intense pain within 30 min to an hour; nausea and vomiting are frequent. There is usually no fever. Rapid resolution of symptoms occurs when the stone is disimpacted. Biliary colic is considered an incorrect use of the term "colic" which is characterized by multiple "waves" of intense pain; proper biliary colic has a single crescendo/decrescendo of pain. Diagnosis is confirmed by abdominal ultrasound. Urgent or elective laparoscopic cholecystectomy is the treatment of choice.

- An impacted stone in the cystic duct may lead to hydrops, empyema, or cholecystitis.
- **Acute cholecystitis,** namely inflammation of the gallbladder, is characterized by the gradual onset of epigastric/RUQ pain which progresses in intensity to its peak. Pain is intense, continuous, unrelenting. It may radiate to the right scapula. Tenderness in the RUQ is characteristic (Murphy's sign). Nausea and vomiting are frequent. There is associated fever. Leukocytosis is present in the labs. Diagnosis is confirmed by abdominal ultrasound. Emergent or urgent (within 72 h) cholecystectomy is the treatment of choice. Laparoscopic cholecystectomy is possible; conversion to open surgery may be needed. In cases of delayed diagnosis, antibiotic treatment may be the initial therapeutic choice. Gallbladder decompression with percutaneous drainage is reserved for cases in which operative therapy is too risky.
- The differential diagnosis of acute cholecystitis includes acute cholangitis, duodenal ulcer, hepatitis, pleurisy, and angina/myocardial infarction.
- Choledocholithiasis occurs when gallstones pass into the extrahepatic ducts. They subsequently may pass into the gastrointestinal system uneventfully, or cause complications such as cholangitis and gallstone pancreatitis.
- Cholangitis is the infection of bile in the extrahepatic ducts as a result of biliary obstruction by stones. Clinically it may manifest similarly to cholecystitis. Charcot's triad (jaundice, pain, and fever) is frequent. In addition to leukocytosis, elevation of direct bilirubin, alkaline phosphatase, and/or γ-glutamyltransferase is observed in the labs. Diagnosis is confirmed by abdominal ultrasound or magnetic cholangiopancreatography (MRCP). Intravenous antibiotics followed by emergent or urgent decompression of the extrahepatic bile ducts with ERCP is the treatment of choice. Other decompressive options are percutaneous transhepatic drainage and operative surgical decompression. The latter carries a high morbidity/mortality rate. Subsequent urgent or elective cholecystectomy is performed.

C. P. Spanos, *Acute Surgical Topics*, https://doi.org/10.1007/978-3-030-68700-7_6

- Gallstone pancreatitis will be discussed in Chap. 7.
- Gallstone ileus is the result of a fistula between the biliary tract (gallbladder, bile duct) and the gastrointestinal tract (stomach, duodenum, small bowel, colon). A gallstone passes through this fistula and most frequently obstructs the terminal ileum. Classic symptoms of small bowel obstruction are manifested. Diagnosis is suggested by plain abdominal films (air in the biliary tree, radiopaque gallstone rarely), CT scan. Abdominal exploration is the treatment of choice (enterotomy, stone extraction). The gallbladder/fistula are usually left alone; the operative morbidity of trying to dissect anatomical structures in this area is high.
- The flora associated with cholecystopathy are Gram-negative aerobes and anaerobes. This is used to guide prophylaxis for surgery, antibiotic treatment for nonoperative therapy, and initial nonoperative therapy for cholangitis.
- Labs utilized in the diagnosis of cholecystopathy are CBC, bilirubin (total, direct and indirect, liver function tests, γ-GT, alkaline phosphatase).
- The most common imaging modality used is abdominal ultrasound. This confirms gallstones, examines the thickness/morphology of gallbladder wall, determines the diameter and contents of the extrahepatic bile ducts. MRCP can depict anatomical details and pathology associated with the bile ducts. CT scans are not the initial imaging modalities of choice; they can detect gallbladder rupture, air in the biliary tree. ERCP is diagnostic and therapeutic for choledocholithiasis/cholangitis.
- Laparoscopic cholecystectomy is one of the commonest surgical procedures performed. The critical view of safety, namely the careful dissection and precise definition of the cystic duct and cystic artery prior to their division are key in this procedure. The difficulty of cholecystectomy increases with inflammation; cholecystectomy within 72 h of onset of cholecystitis is recommended. Injury to the extrahepatic bile ducts and major vascular structures causes significant morbidity and mortality and is more common with inflammation.

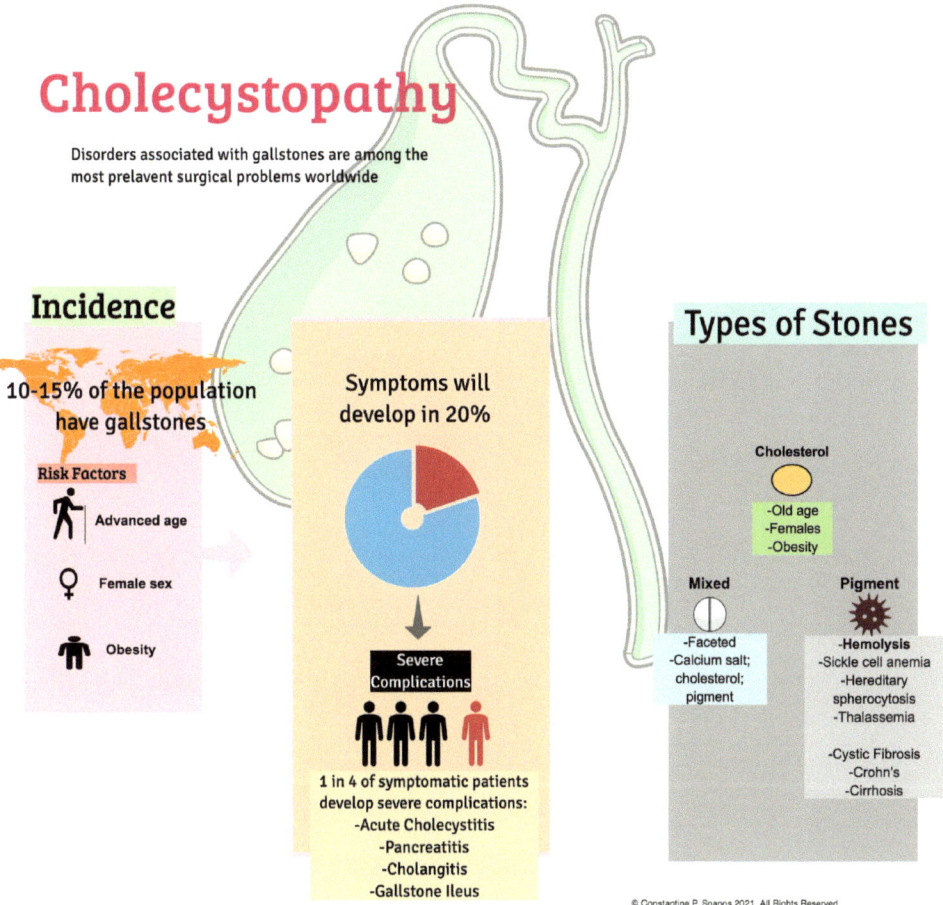

Cholecystopathy

Disorders associated with gallstones are among the most prelavent surgical problems worldwide

Incidence

10-15% of the population have gallstones

Risk Factors

Advanced age

Female sex

Obesity

Symptoms will develop in 20%

Severe Complications

1 in 4 of symptomatic patients develop severe complications:
-Acute Cholecystitis
-Pancreatitis
-Cholangitis
-Gallstone Ileus

Types of Stones

Cholesterol
-Old age
-Females
-Obesity

Mixed
-Faceted
-Calcium salt; cholesterol; pigment

Pigment
-Hemolysis
-Sickle cell anemia
-Hereditary spherocytosis
-Thalassemia

-Cystic Fibrosis
-Crohn's
-Cirrhosis

Cholecystopathy

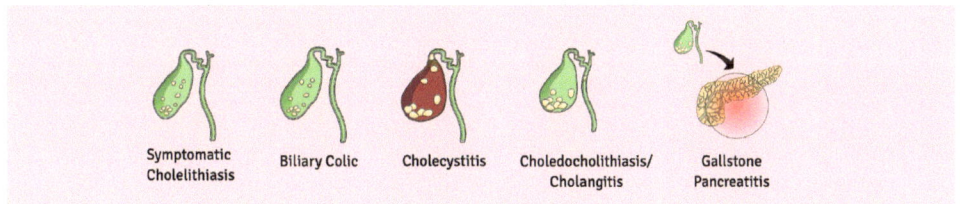

Symptomatic Cholelithiasis | Biliary Colic | Cholecystitis | Choledocholithiasis/Cholangitis | Gallstone Pancreatitis

Each condition has a distinctive clinical pattern. A careful history and physical exam leads to diagnosis in most cases.

Imaging supplements the history & physical; usually is confirmatory

Clinical Manifestation

Cholecystopathy may manifest in any one of these conditions. There are no predictive factors regarding the modality of the initial attack.

In addition, recurrent attacks are also unpredictable regarding modality and severity.

In order of decreased to increased severity (morbidity) one can classify cholecystopathy as follows:

-Symptomatic cholelithiasis
-Bilary colic
-Cholecystitis
-Gallstone pancreatitis
-Cholangitis

Symptomatic cholelithiasis

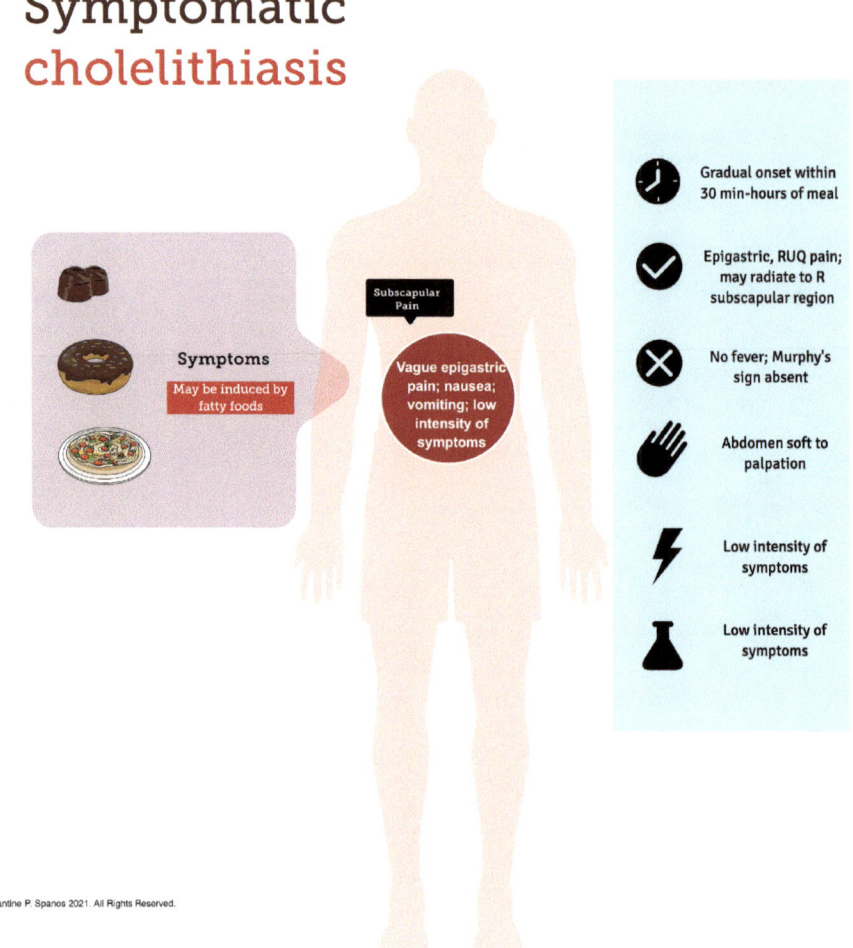

Symptoms

May be induced by fatty foods

Subscapular Pain

Vague epigastric pain; nausea; vomiting; low intensity of symptoms

Gradual onset within 30 min-hours of meal

Epigastric, RUQ pain; may radiate to R subscapular region

No fever; Murphy's sign absent

Abdomen soft to palpation

Low intensity of symptoms

Low intensity of symptoms

Biliary Colic

Common manifestation of acute abdomen. Frequent manifestation of cholecystopathy.

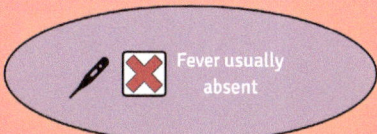 Fever usually absent

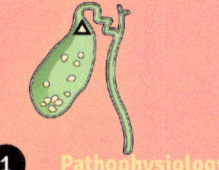

1 Pathophysiology

Intermittent obstruction of cystic duct/gallbladder neck; gallbladder contraction against obstruction causes symptoms

2 Onset and timing of pain

Severe pain within 30 min/hours; usually after meal; may wake from sleep

 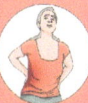

3 Pain radiation/associated symptoms

Pain may radiate to right subscapular region or lower back; Nausea/vomiting present; concomitant with pain

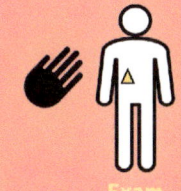

4 Exam

Soft abdominal wall; tender on deep palaption in RUQ; not quite Murphy's sign

5 Labs

Usually normal; leukocytosis infrequent

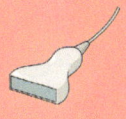

6 Imaging

Ultrasound sensitive/specific; gallstones detected; no gallbladder wall thichening; always make an effort to visualize common bile duct/hepatic bile ducts to assess dilatation

Colic vs Cholecystitis

In colic there is a pain 'peak and trough'; in cholecystitis there is a gradual increase in pain intensity, becoming continuous and unrelenting subsequently

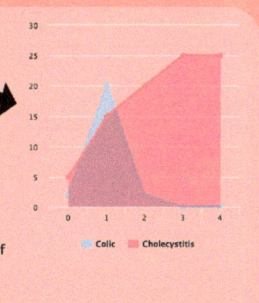

Antibiotics

May be indicated in cholecystitis; not in colic

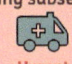

Urgent Surgery

Ideally, within 72 hours after cholecystitis is diagnosed

Elective Surgery

Appropriate in biliary colic; if surgery is not performed urgently in cholecystitis, elective surgery after 6-8 weeks is indicated; however, recurrence risk is high

Stone Impaction

Gallstones impacted at gallbladder neck or the cystic duct may lead to the following:

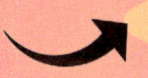

Hydrops

Bile pigment and bile salts get reabsorbed by gallbladder mucosa; white and mucous fluid accumulates

Empyema

When bacteria invade cystic bile, fluid becomes purulent; bacteria are usually spread through the hematogenous route

Acute Cholecystitis

Inflammation of gallbladder wall due to several causes: mucosal injury from stones; ischemia due to increased intraluminal pressure; bacterial invasion

Cholecystitis

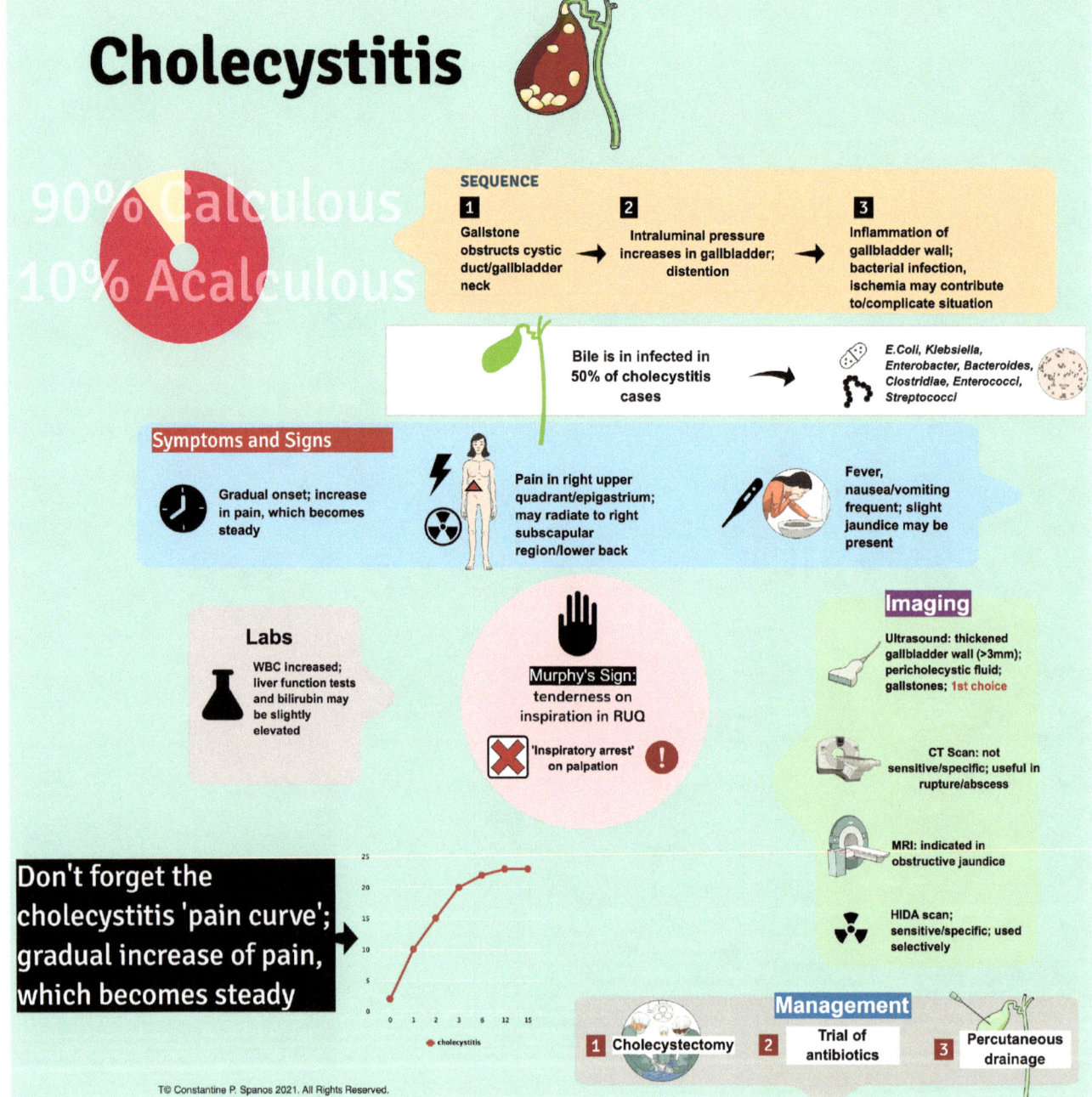

90% Calculous
10% Acalculous

SEQUENCE

1 Gallstone obstructs cystic duct/gallbladder neck → **2** Intraluminal pressure increases in gallbladder; distention → **3** Inflammation of gallbladder wall; bacterial infection, ischemia may contribute to/complicate situation

Bile is in infected in 50% of cholecystitis cases → E.Coli, Klebsiella, Enterobacter, Bacteroides, Clostridiae, Enterococci, Streptococci

Symptoms and Signs

Gradual onset; increase in pain, which becomes steady

Pain in right upper quadrant/epigastrium; may radiate to right subscapular region/lower back

Fever, nausea/vomiting frequent; slight jaundice may be present

Labs

WBC increased; liver function tests and bilirubin may be slightly elevated

Murphy's Sign: tenderness on inspiration in RUQ

'Inspiratory arrest' on palpation

Imaging

Ultrasound: thickened gallbladder wall (>3mm); pericholecystic fluid; gallstones; 1st choice

CT Scan: not sensitive/specific; useful in rupture/abscess

MRI: indicated in obstructive jaundice

HIDA scan; sensitive/specific; used selectively

Don't forget the cholecystitis 'pain curve'; gradual increase of pain, which becomes steady

◆ cholecystitis

Management

1 Cholecystectomy **2** Trial of antibiotics **3** Percutaneous drainage

Differential Diagnosis/Cholecystitis

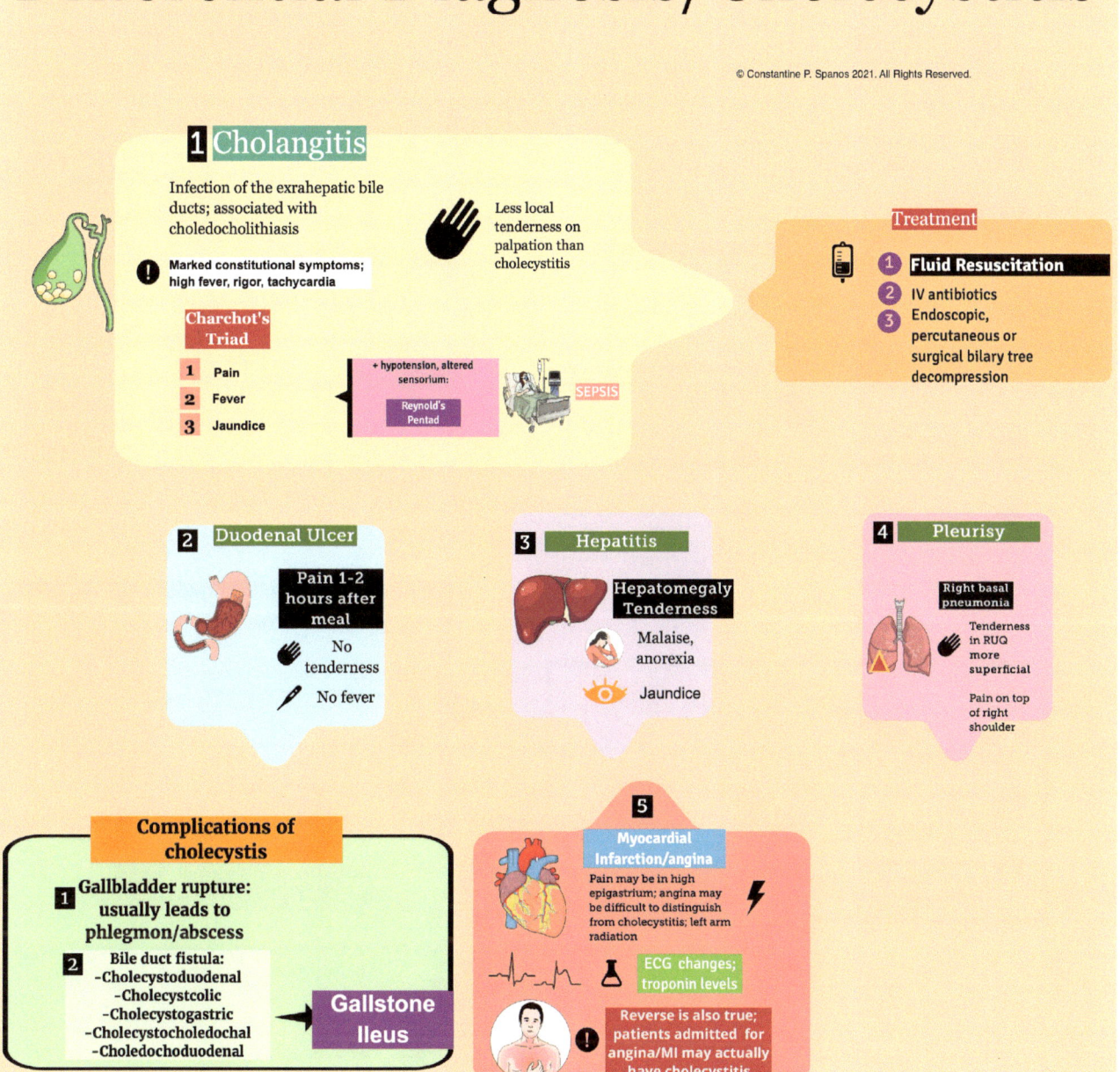

1 Cholangitis

Infection of the exrahepatic bile ducts; associated with choledocholithiasis

Less local tenderness on palpation than cholecystitis

Marked constitutional symptoms; high fever, rigor, tachycardia

Charchot's Triad

1 Pain
2 Fever
3 Jaundice

+ hypotension, altered sensorium:

Reynold's Pentad

SEPSIS

Treatment

1 **Fluid Resuscitation**
2 IV antibiotics
3 Endoscopic, percutaneous or surgical bilary tree decompression

2 Duodenal Ulcer

Pain 1-2 hours after meal

No tenderness

No fever

3 Hepatitis

Hepatomegaly Tenderness

Malaise, anorexia

Jaundice

4 Pleurisy

Right basal pneumonia

Tenderness in RUQ more superficial

Pain on top of right shoulder

Complications of cholecystis

1 Gallbladder rupture: usually leads to phlegmon/abscess

2 Bile duct fistula:
-Cholecystoduodenal
-Cholecystcolic
-Cholecystogastric
-Cholecystocholedochal
-Choledochoduodenal

Gallstone Ileus

5 Myocardial Infarction/angina

Pain may be in high epigastrium; angina may be difficult to distinguish from cholecystitis; left arm radiation

ECG changes; troponin levels

Reverse is also true; patients admitted for angina/MI may actually have cholecystitis

Cholecystopathy: treatment

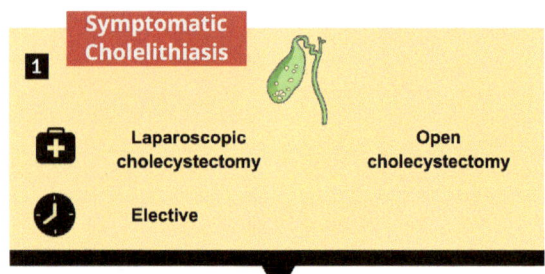

Symptomatic Cholelithiasis

1

- Laparoscopic cholecystectomy
- Open cholecystectomy
- Elective

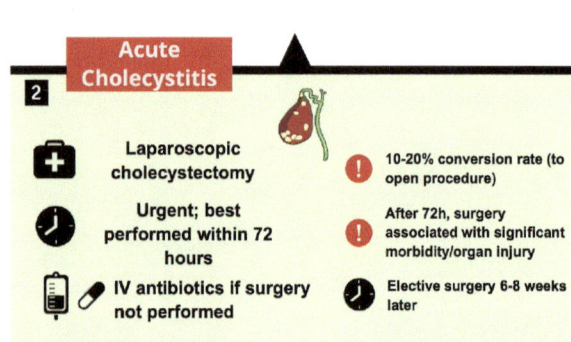

Acute Cholecystitis

2

- Laparoscopic cholecystectomy
- Urgent; best performed within 72 hours
- IV antibiotics if surgery not performed

- ! 10-20% conversion rate (to open procedure)
- ! After 72h, surgery associated with significant morbidity/organ injury
- Elective surgery 6-8 weeks later

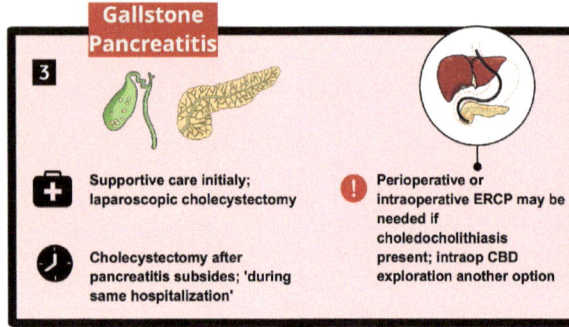

Gallstone Pancreatitis

3

- Supportive care initialy; laparoscopic cholecystectomy
- Cholecystectomy after pancreatitis subsides; 'during same hospitalization'

- ! Perioperative or intraoperative ERCP may be needed if choledocholithiasis present; intraop CBD exploration another option

Laparoscopic Cholecystectomy

Standard of care; allows for quick recovery, less pain, better quality of life; dissection using **critical view of safety** important, since there are anatomic variations

Conversion rate (to open procedure) < 1%; complications include cystic duct stump leak; common bile duct injury; conversion rate greater with cholecystitis (10-20%)

Contraindications to laparoscopy include inability to tolerate carboperitoneum; unsafe dissection; bleeding; major injury

Steps

- Carboperitoneum
- Critical view of safety dissection
- Cystic duct ligation/division
- Cystic artery ligation/division

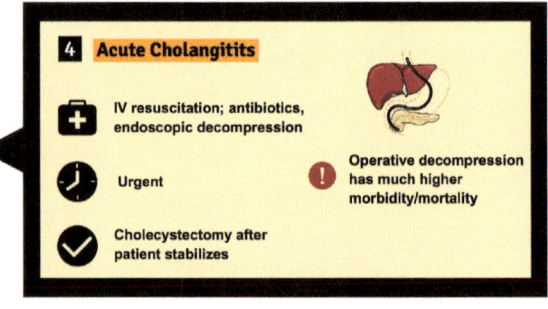

4 **Acute Cholangitits**

- IV resuscitation; antibiotics, endoscopic decompression
- Urgent
- Cholecystectomy after patient stabilizes

- ! Operative decompression has much higher morbidity/mortality

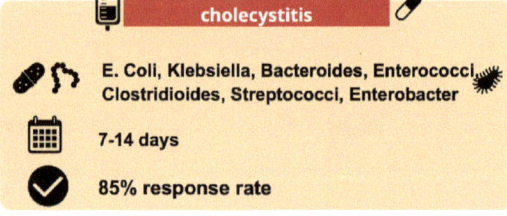

Antibiotics in acute cholecystitis

- E. Coli, Klebsiella, Bacteroides, Enterococci Clostridioides, Streptococci, Enterobacter
- 7-14 days
- 85% response rate

Prophylactic Cholecystectomy

Asymptomatic cholelithiasis is usually managed expectantly; however there are certain clinical conditions and disorders in which prophylactic cholecystectomy may be considered

Gallblladder Polyps

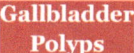

Usually asymptomatic; size > 1cm indication for cholecystectomy

Gastrectomy/Gastric cancer

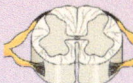

Lithogenesis as a result of:
-Sympathetic/parasympathetic denervation
-Duodenal exclusion (↓ CCK)
-Rapid weight loss
-Biliary stasis

Concomitant cholecystectomy recommended

Transplantation

-Increased incidence prevalence of gallstones in transplant patients
-Increased morbidity/mortality with emergency cholecystectomy/biliary sepsis

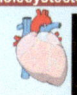

Prophylactic cholecystectomy in heart/kidney transplant recipients

Spinal cord injury

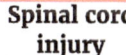

-30% incidence of gallstones in spinal cord injury
-22% incidence of complications of gallstones

Gallbladder wall calcifications

-Focal calcifications (focal depositis, selective mucosal calcifications

-Diffuse intramural calcification (Porcelain gallbladder)

-Focal calcifications at higher risk for malignancy (25% vs 16% in diffuse calcification)

Hemoglobinopathy

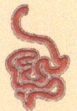

-Sickle cell disease: 70% incidence of cholelithiasis
Adulthood: high rate of progression to symptomatic disease

-Herediatry spherocytosis: cholecystectomy + splenectomy

Extensive small bowel resection

-Short gut syndrome
-Altered enterohepatic cycle
-Carcinoid syndrome secondary to chronic somatostatin analogue administration

Somatostatin: 63% develop gallstones

Bariatric Surgery

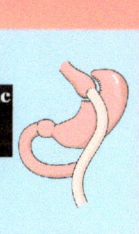

30% incidence of symptomatic gallstones post bariatric surgery

Ursodiol treatment for prophylaxis: decreses gallstone incidence to 8%

Further Reading

Bile duct fistulae. In: Reynolds JC, Ward PJ, Martin JA, Su GL, Whitcomb DC, editors. The Netter collection of medical illustrations digestive system: Part III-Liver, biliary tract, and pancreas, vol 9. 2nd ed. Philadelphia: Elsevier; 2017. p. 124.

Chen CC, Chapman WC. Surgical diseases of the biliary tree. In: Klingensmith ME, Vemuri C, Fayanju OM, Robertson JO, Samson JO, Sanford D, editors. The Washington manual of surgery. 7th ed. Philadelphia: Wolters Kluwer; 2016. p. 372–87.

Fagenholz PJ, Velmahos GC. The management of acute cholecystitis. In: Cameron JL, Cameron AM, editors. Current surgical therapy. 12th ed. Philadelphia: Elsevier; 2017. p. 430–3.

Gall bladder stones. In: McLatchie G, Borley N, Chikwe J, editors. Oxford handbook of clinical surgery. 4th ed. Oxford: Oxford University Press; 2013. p. 316–317.

Hydrops and empyema of gallbladder. In: Reynolds JC, Ward PJ, Martin JA, Su GL, Whitcomb DC, editors. The Netter collection of medical illustrations digestive system: Part III-Liver, biliary tract, and pancreas, vol 9. 2nd ed. Philadelphia: Elsevier; 2017. p. 119.

Silen W. Cholecystitis and other causes of acute pain in the right upper quadrant of the abdomen. In: Silen W, editor. Cope's early diagnosis of the acute abdomen. 22nd ed. New York: Oxford University Press; 2010. p. 131–40.

- Acute pancreatitis is a disorder of variable clinical severity. As a result of a cascade of released cytokines as well as pancreatic enzymes, it can be self-limiting with mild clinical symptoms, or severe with leading to systemic inflammatory reaction syndrome (SIRS) and multi-organ dysfunction syndrome (MODS).
- Etiologies of pancreatitis include:
  - Gallstones (60%)
  - Alcohol consumption (30%)
  - Hyperlipidemia
  - Venom (snake/scorpion)
  - Drugs (azathioprine, estrogen, thiazides, steroids, NSAIDS)
  - Hypercalcemia (hyperparathyroidism, multiple myeloma)
  - Infection (CMV, mumps, hepatitis B, mycoplasma)
  - Direct pancreatic injury (ERCP, trauma, surgery, coronary bypass)
  - Idiopathic
- Pathologically, pancreatitis can be classified as edematous (70%), necrotizing (25%), and hemorrhagic (5%)
- Several disease severity scoring systems are utilized for pancreatitis. The Glasgow-Imrie Scale and the Ranson Criteria use age and laboratory values to predict severity. The CTSI (Computed tomography severity index) uses pancreatic morphology, extent of pancreatic necrosis, and extrapancreatic lesions as depicted on CT to predict severity.
- The systemic inflammatory response in pancreatitis may cause deleterious effects in intravascular volume, renal perfusion as well as alveolar injury. Pulmonary complications occur in approximately 50% of cases of severe pancreatitis. ARDS confers high mortality.
- Patients with pancreatitis have a history of progressive onset of epigastric pain, which increases in intensity and is continuous. The pain may radiate to the back. Nausea and vomiting are common and may be severe. Fever is not uncommon. In severe cases, patients have tachycardia, tachypnea, and hypotension. On physical exam patients appear unwell and anxious. Signs of hypovolemia may be present. There may be reduced breath sounds on auscultation. Tenderness to deep palpation in the entire abdomen is common. Periumbilical (Cullen's sign) and flank (Grey-Turner sign) ecchymoses, classically described in hemorrhagic pancreatitis, are rare.
- The immediate management of patients with acute pancreatitis includes:
  - Assessment of ABCs (airway, breathing, circulation)
  - Supplemental oxygen
  - Adequate IV access
  - Crystalloid fluid resuscitation
  - Hemodynamic, oxygen monitoring, including Foley catheter placement
  - Nasogastric decompression if vomiting is severe
- Labs are obtained: CBC, electrolytes, BUN/creatinine, liver function tests, albumin, LDH, calcium, and ABG's. These may be used to formulate the severity scores mentioned previously. Of note, serum amylase and lipase, used for laboratory confirmation of pancreatitis, are not included in these severity scores!
- Imaging in pancreatitis is important in confirmation of diagnosis and classification of pathological type as well as severity of the disease. The CT scan is the most frequently used modality. It is recommended that in most cases imaging should be obtained at 48 h after onset of symptoms or admission; delineation of pancreatic pathology is considered superior at this juncture. An abdominal ultrasound should always be obtained to confirm the presence of gallstones. MRCP is performed when there is suspicion of choledocholithiasis or other biliary obstructive etiologies.
- Principles of care in acute pancreatitis are in essence **optimized multisystemic support** and include:
  - Volume resuscitation. The goal is a urinary output of 0.5 ml/kg/h; avoid fluid overload.
  - Bowel rest. Tube enteral feeds are preferable to TPN.
  - Respiratory monitoring and support. Oxygen therapy as needed.
  - Antibiotics are indicated for confirmed active infection (UTI, cholangitis, pneumonia, bacteremia, catheter

infection, infected pancreatic necrosis). Prophylactic antibiotics are no longer recommended.

- – Critical care/ICU. The goal is maintenance of normal hemodynamics and end-organ perfusion. Vasopressors and ventilatory support are given as needed.
- – Indications for surgical care include clinical deterioration despite best supportive care, worsening sepsis, and bleeding, perforation. Pancreatic debridement, the indicated surgical procedure, is best delayed to allow for sequestration of necrosis (18–20 days). After resolution of an episode of gallbladder pancreatitis, cholecystectomy should be performed, ideally during the same hospitalization.

- Complications of acute pancreatitis include pseudocysts, infected pancreatic necrosis, and visceral pseudoaneurysms.
- Pseudocysts result from pancreatic duct disruption and form within 4 weeks of an attack of acute pancreatitis. Non-symptomatic pseudocysts are managed conservatively. Symptomatic pseudocysts, or those complicated by infection, hemorrhage, obstruction, or rupture, are managed by interventional radiology, endoscopy, or surgery.
- Infected pancreatic necrosis is a complication of necrotizing pancreatitis in 5–10% of cases. The diagnosis is made by CT (air in necrotic pancreatic parenchyma). Subsequent percutaneous FNA/blood culture depicting flora are confirmatory to the diagnosis. Treatment includes percutaneous/endoscopic drainage or laparoscopic/open surgical debridement.
- Visceral pseudoaneurysms occur in the splenic, left gastric, and gastroduodenal artery. Rupture may lead to hemosuccus pancreaticus and/or hemorrhagic shock. Treatment includes arterial embolization by interventional radiology, and surgery.

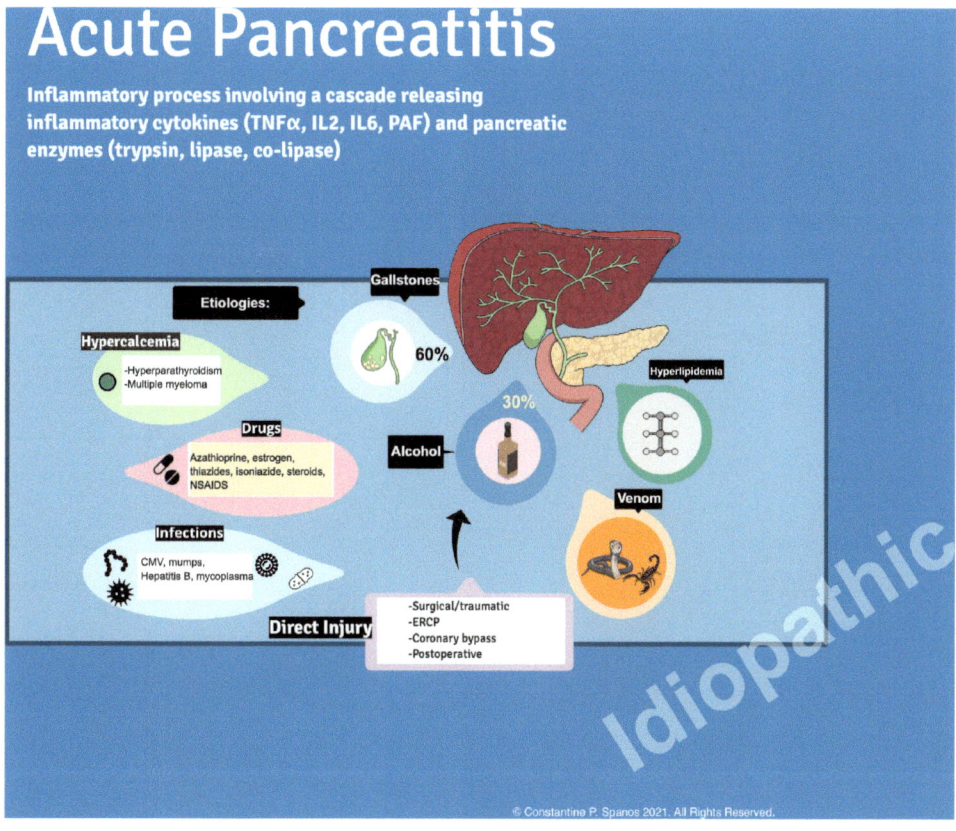

Classification, Assessment, Initial Management of Pancreatitis

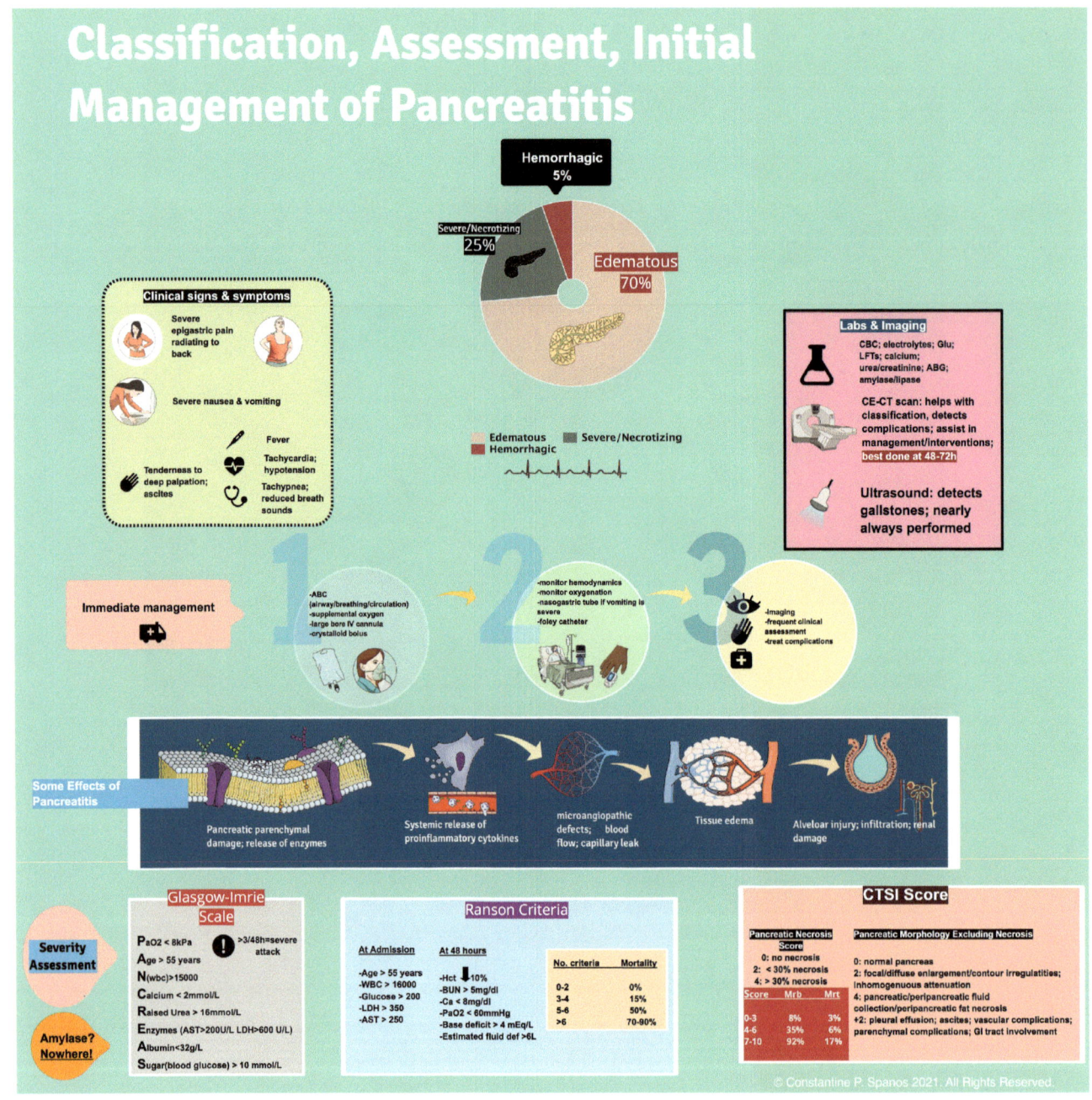

Hemorrhagic 5%

Severe/Necrotizing 25%

Edematous 70%

Edematous   Severe/Necrotizing
Hemorrhagic

Clinical signs & symptoms
- Severe epigastric pain radiating to back
- Severe nausea & vomiting
- Fever
- Tachycardia; hypotension
- Tenderness to deep palpation; ascites
- Tachypnea; reduced breath sounds

Labs & Imaging
CBC; electrolytes; Glu; LFTs; calcium; urea/creatinine; ABG; amylase/lipase

CE-CT scan: helps with classification, detects complications; assist in management/interventions; best done at 48-72h

Ultrasound: detects gallstones; nearly always performed

Immediate management

1
-ABC (airway/breathing/circulation)
-supplemental oxygen
-large bore IV cannula
-crystalloid bolus

2
-monitor hemodynamics
-monitor oxygenation
-nasogastric tube if vomiting is severe
-foley catheter

3
-Imaging
-frequent clinical assessment
-treat complications

Some Effects of Pancreatitis
- Pancreatic parenchymal damage; release of enzymes
- Systemic release of proinflammatory cytokines
- microangiopathic defects; blood flow; capillary leak
- Tissue edema
- Alveolar injury; infiltration; renal damage

Glasgow-Imrie Scale

Severity Assessment

P$_{aO2}$ < 8kPa   >3/48h=severe attack
A$_{ge}$ > 55 years
N$_{(wbc)}$>15000
C$_{alcium}$ < 2mmol/L
R$_{aised}$ Urea > 16mmol/L
E$_{nzymes}$ (AST>200U/L LDH>600 U/L)
A$_{lbumin}$<32g/L
S$_{ugar}$(blood glucose) > 10 mmol/L

Amylase? Nowhere!

Ranson Criteria

At Admission
-Age > 55 years
-WBC > 16000
-Glucose > 200
-LDH > 350
-AST > 250

At 48 hours
-Hct ↓10%
-BUN > 5mg/dl
-Ca < 8mg/dl
-PaO2 < 60mmHg
-Base deficit > 4 mEq/L
-Estimated fluid def >6L

No. criteria	Mortality
0-2	0%
3-4	15%
5-6	50%
>6	70-90%

CTSI Score

Pancreatic Necrosis Score
0: no necrosis
2: < 30% necrosis
4: > 30% necrosis

Score	Mrb	Mrt
0-3	8%	3%
4-6	35%	6%
7-10	92%	17%

Pancreatic Morphology Excluding Necrosis
0: normal pancreas
2: focal/diffuse enlargement/contour irregularities; inhomogenuous attenuation
4: pancreatic/peripancreatic fluid collection/peripancreatic fat necrosis
+2: pleural effusion; ascites; vascular complications; parenchymal complications; GI tract involvement

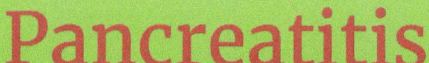

Pancreatitis

Pancreatitis is a disorder that has variable severity. The inflammation may be self-limited with mild clinical symptoms; however, it may be severe with significant systemic involvement resulting in dysfunction of many organs. Treatment is usually supportive; most organ systems must be diligently assesed and traeted accordingly.

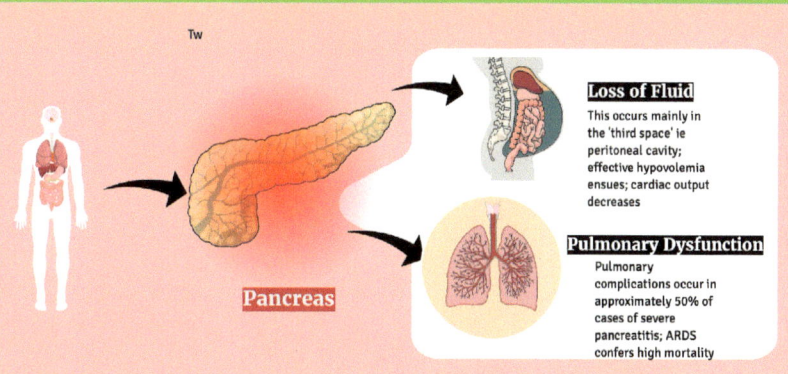

Tw

Pancreas

Loss of Fluid
This occurs mainly in the 'third space' ie peritoneal cavity; effective hypovolemia ensues; cardiac output decreases

Pulmonary Dysfunction
Pulmonary complications occur in approximately 50% of cases of severe pancreatitis; ARDS confers high mortality

Principles of care:

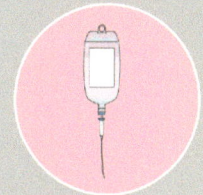

1 Volume Resuscitation

-Isotonic fluids
-Avoid overload (pulmonary edema/ARDS/compartment syndrome)
-Urinary output: 0.5ml/kg/h

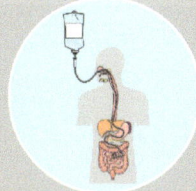

2 Bowel Rest

-Nasogastric tube if vomiting severe
-Enteral feeding preferable to parenteral; decreased infection rates/surgical interventions/LOS

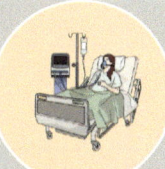

3 Respiratory Monitoring & Support

-Assess oxygenation
- Supportive care/oxygen therapy
-ABG if clinical deterioration
-Assess acid/base status
rates/surgical interventions/LOS

4 Antibiotics

-Indicated for underlined confirmed active infection
- Broad spectrum/Gram -/fungi
-Prophylactic antibiotics NOT recommended

-UTI
-Cholangitis
-Pneumonia
-Catheter infection
-Bacteremia
-INFECTED PANCREATIC NECROSIS

5 Surgical Care Indications:

-Clinical deterioration
- Sepsis
-Bleeding
-Perforation
-PANCREATIC DEBRIDEMENT: best delayed to allow for sequestration of necrosis (18-20 days)

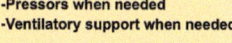

6 Critical Care

-Maintain normal hemodynamics
-Maintain end organ perfusion
-Pressors when needed
-Ventilatory support when needed

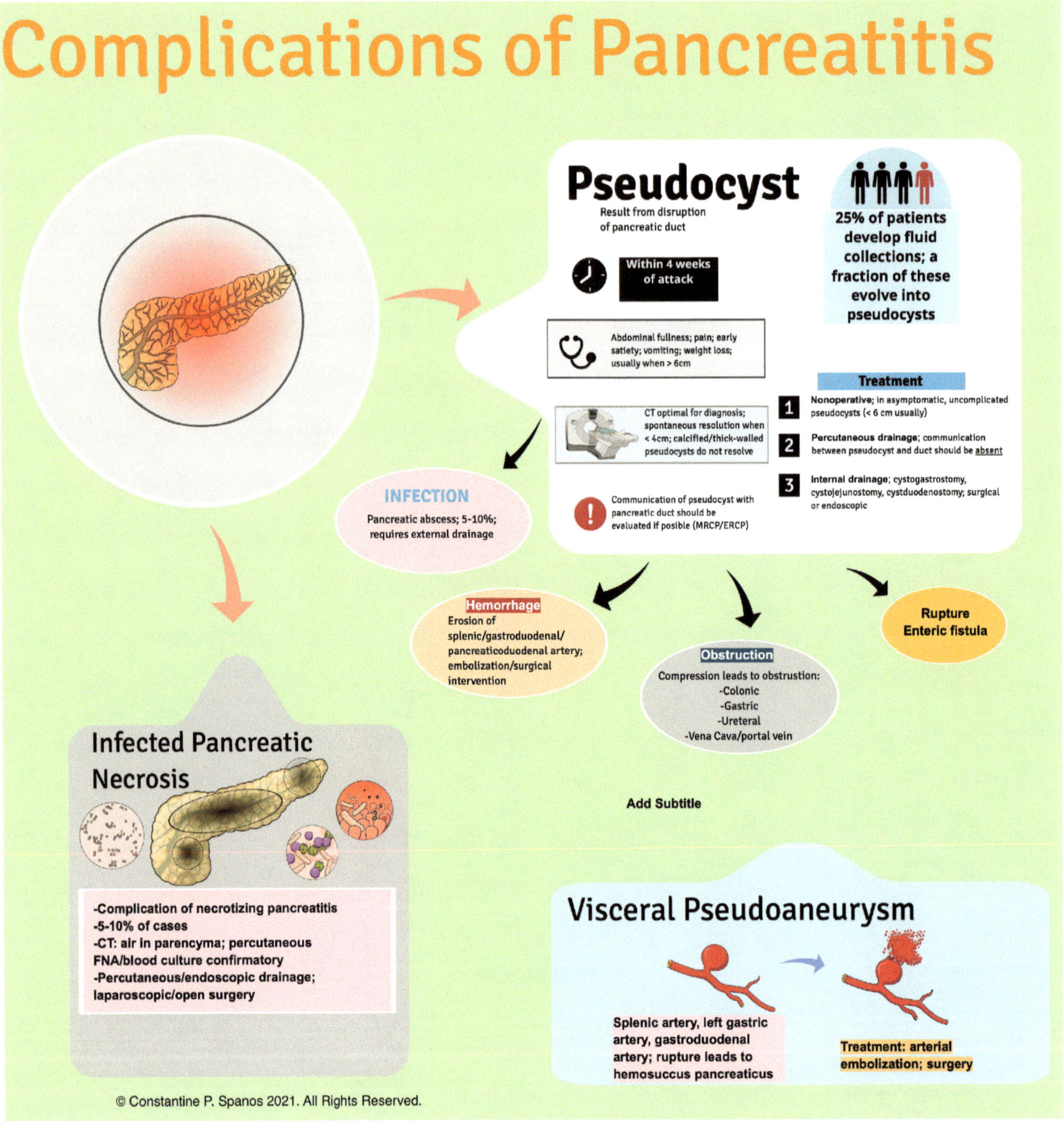

Complications of Pancreatitis

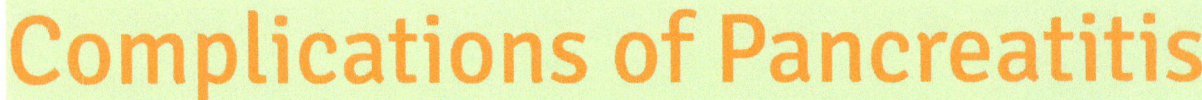

Pseudocyst

Result from disruption
of pancreatic duct

**Within 4 weeks
of attack**

Abdominal fullness; pain; early
satiety; vomiting; weight loss;
usually when > 6cm

CT optimal for diagnosis;
spontaneous resolution when
< 4cm; calcified/thick-walled
pseudocysts do not resolve

Communication of pseudocyst with
pancreatic duct should be
evaluated if posible (MRCP/ERCP)

**25% of patients
develop fluid
collections; a
fraction of these
evolve into
pseudocysts**

Treatment

1 Nonoperative; in asymptomatic, uncomplicated
pseudocysts (< 6 cm usually)

2 Percutaneous drainage; communication
between pseudocyst and duct should be <u>absent</u>

3 Internal drainage; cystogastrostomy,
cystojejunostomy, cystduodenostomy; surgical
or endoscopic

INFECTION

Pancreatic abscess; 5-10%;
requires external drainage

Hemorrhage
Erosion of
splenic/gastroduodenal/
pancreaticoduodenal artery;
embolization/surgical
intervention

Obstruction
Compression leads to obstrustion:
-Colonic
-Gastric
-Ureteral
-Vena Cava/portal vein

**Rupture
Enteric fistula**

Add Subtitle

Infected Pancreatic Necrosis

-Complication of necrotizing pancreatitis
-5-10% of cases
-CT: air in parencyma; percutaneous
FNA/blood culture confirmatory
-Percutaneous/endoscopic drainage;
laparoscopic/open surgery

Visceral Pseudoaneurysm

Splenic artery, left gastric
artery, gastroduodenal
artery; rupture leads to
hemosuccus pancreaticus

**Treatment: arterial
embolization; surgery**

Further Reading

Acute pancreatitis. In: McLatchie G, Borley N, Chikwe J, editors. Oxford handbook of clinical surgery. 4th ed. Oxford: Oxford University Press; 2013. p. 332–5.

LaFace A, Davis D, Velanovich V. The management of acute pancreatitis. In: Cameron JL, Cameron AM, editors. Current surgical therapy. 12th ed. Philadelphia: Elsevier; 2017. p. 489–92.

Sanford DE, Strasberg SM. Surgical diseases of the pancreas. In: Klingensmith ME, Vemuri C, Fayanju OM, Robertson JO, Samson JO, Sanford D, editors. The Washington manual of surgery. 7th ed. Philadelphia: Wolters Kluwer; 2016. p. 388–406.

Silen W. Acute pancreatitis. In: Silen W, editor. Cope's early diagnosis of the acute abdomen. 22nd ed. New York: Oxford University Press; 2010. p. 122–30.

- Diverticular disease is the most common benign condition of the colon. Diverticula are outpouchings of the colonic mucosa/submucosa through interruptions of the muscular layer associated with small arteries supplying the mucosa. The prevalent etiopathogenic theory for diverticular formation is that of chronically increased colonic intraluminal pressure resulting from a low-fiber, Western type diet.
- The frequency of diverticular formation increases with age. In western populations, the sigmoid colon is affected most frequently. In far-eastern populations, right-sided diverticulosis is more prevalent. In addition, the incidence of diverticular disease has increased in populations which have adopted a western type diet.
- The two manifestations of diverticular disease are acute diverticulitis and diverticular bleeding. **Diverticulosis** is the mere presence of (usually multiple) diverticula.
- Acute diverticulitis will develop in 20% of individuals with diverticulosis.
- After a single attack of acute diverticulitis, there is a 10–20% chance of a second attack. Patients with a history of two attacks have a 40–60% chance of a third attack.
- Clinically, acute diverticulitis presents with gradual onset of left-sided abdominal pain. Pain is continuous; may be associated with constipation or diarrhea, and fever is frequent. On examination, tenderness is elicited upon palpation in the hypogastrium/LLQ. Disease in patients with a redundant sigmoid colon may present with RLQ pain and tenderness, mimicking appendicitis. Patients with free perforation or a ruptured diverticular abscess present with diffuse peritonitis.
- Complications of acute diverticulitis include abscess formation, free perforation, stenosis, and fistulization. Colovesical fistulae are most common.
- Laboratory evaluation reveals leukocytosis with a left shift.
- Plain abdominal films can show free air with perforation. CT scan with triple contrast is useful to confirm the diagnosis and classify the disease. CT imaging can also be used to guide abscess drainage.
- The Modified Hinchey Classification is commonly used:
  - Hinchey 0: Mild symptomatology, ±fever, with few, if any, findings on CT
  - Hinchey Ia: Confined pericolic inflammation/phlegmon on CT
  - Hinchey Ib: Confined pericolic abscess on CT
  - Hinchey II: Pelvic/distant/peritoneal abscess on CT
  - Hinchey III: Purulent peritonitis
  - Hinchey IV: Feculent peritonitis
- Hinchey 0 is frequently termed SUDD (symptomatic uncomplicated diverticular disease). This term is not widely accepted; it may be confused with irritable bowel syndrome (IBS).
- The treatment for acute diverticulitis includes treatment with or without antibiotics, interventional radiological procedures, minimally invasive or open surgery with or without resection, with or without creation of a stoma.
- Uncomplicated diverticulitis (Hinchey 0/SUDD-Ia) is conventionally treated with PO/IV antibiotics and bowel rest until symptoms resolve. Recent studies have shown that treatment without antibiotics may have similar outcomes.
- Patients with small abscesses (<4 cm) may be treated with antibiotics; these usually resolve without intervention. Larger abscesses can be drained under CT guidance. Inability to drain with this modality mandates surgical intervention.
- The recurrence rate after abscess resolution is 40%.
- Planned resection may follow abscess resolution. Mandatory resection is currently under debate.
- Currently, individualized treatment is recommended for acute diverticulitis. Attack frequency, severity, and quality of life are considered for surgical intervention.
- Colonoscopy is recommended after resolution of acute diverticulitis, to rule out malignancy (1% incidence).
- Patients with peritonitis are treated surgically. Purulent and fecal peritonitis are **operative** diagnoses.

C. P. Spanos, *Acute Surgical Topics*, https://doi.org/10.1007/978-3-030-68700-7_8

- **Elective surgical procedures (open, laparoscopic/robotic)**:
  - Primary resection and anastomosis. The diseased portion of the bowel is resected; anastomosis should not have ischemia, tension, and/or diverticula! Sound surgical technique is paramount.
  - A stoma is rarely required.
  - Colovesical fistulas are usually dealt with by "pinching off" the diseased colon from the bladder. Primary closure of bladder defect is not mandatory. A Foley catheter is left in place for 7–10 days.
- **Urgent/emergent procedures** (open, laparoscopic, robotic):
  - Primary resection with anastomosis. Healthy bowel is required for anastomosis. A diverting ileostomy/colostomy may be fashioned.
  - Hartmann's procedure. This remains the most commonly performed emergent procedure for acute diverticulitis. It has high operative morbidity and stoma non-reversal rate.
  - Laparoscopic lavage without resection has been used in cases of purulent peritonitis. Studies have demonstrated a lower rate of stoma creation/resection. It is not considered standard of care and is under debate.

Diverticular Disease

Diverticular disease is the most frequent benign condition of the colon. Diverticula are outpouchings of the colonic mucosa/submucosa through interruptions of the muscular layer associated with small arteries supplying the mucosa.

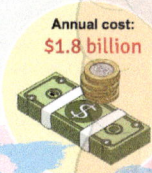

Annual cost:
$1.8 billion

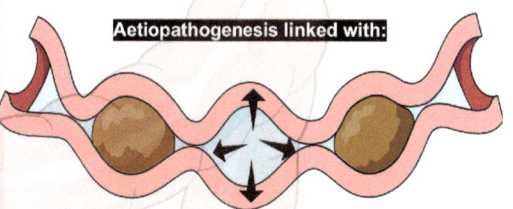

Aetiopathogenesis linked with:

Increased colonic intraluminal pressure

Western Societies

USA
300,000 admissions/y

Frequency of diverticulae increase with age; after 50: follows age; i.e. 80% in people of 80 years

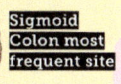
Sigmoid Colon most frequent site

Far East

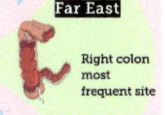
Right colon most frequent site

In countries which have adopted a Western diet, incidence of diverticular disease has increased

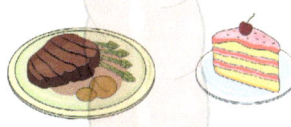

Low-fiber diet

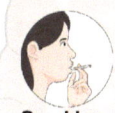

Smoking

Sequelae of diverticulosis

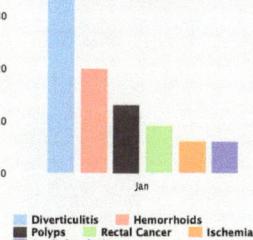

Causes of lower GI bleeding (%)

(bar chart, y-axis 0–40, labeled "Jan")

Legend:
- Diverticulitis
- Hemorrhoids
- Polyps
- Rectal Cancer
- Ischemia
- Angiodysplasia

1 Low GI Bleeding

Diverticulosis is one of the most frequent causes of massive (> 2U PRBC/24h) lower gastrointestinal bleeding.

Bleeding stops spontaneously in 80% of cases; recurs (requiring intervention) in 25% of cases

2 Diverticulitis

Inflammation
Abscess
Purulent peritonitis
Fecal peritonitis
Fistulization

20% of individuals with diverticulosis will develop diverticulitis

20% Diverticulitis

80% Asymtomatic

Diverticulitis   Asymptomatic

Patients with one attack of diverticultis have a 10-20% chance of a second attack

Patients with a history of two attacks have a 40-60% cance of a third attack

Diverticulitis

Colonic wall inflammation secondary to stasis within diverticulum. Microperforation/macroperforation may lead to phlegmon, abscess formation and peritonitis

Symptoms/Presentation

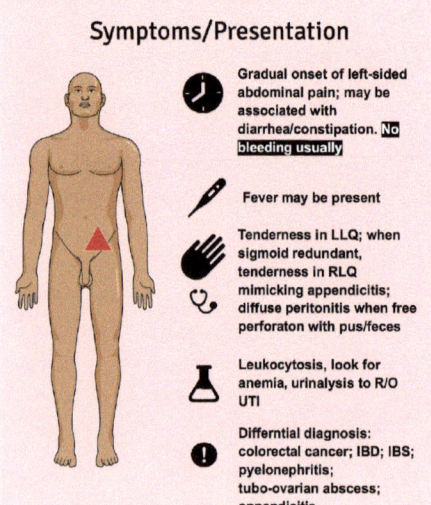

🕐 Gradual onset of left-sided abdominal pain; may be associated with diarrhea/constipation. **No bleeding usually**

🌡 Fever may be present

✋ Tenderness in LLQ; when sigmoid redundant, tenderness in RLQ mimicking appendicitis; diffuse peritonitis when free perforaton with pus/feces

🧪 Leukocytosis, look for anemia, urinalysis to R/O UTI

❗ Differntial diagnosis: colorectal cancer; IBD; IBS; pyelonephritis; tubo-ovarian abscess; appendicitis

Imaging

☢ **Plain abdominal films:** look for free air; constipation; colonic distention

CT scan: triple contrast ideal (PO/IV/rectal); helps classify diverticulitis

Fistula from diverticulitis

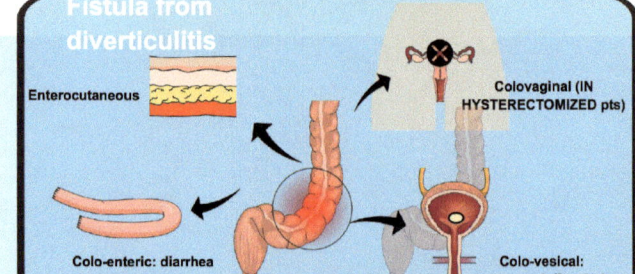

Enterocutaneous

Colovaginal (IN HYSTERECTOMIZED pts)

Colo-enteric: diarrhea

Colo-vesical: pneumaturia/fecaluria

Modified Hinchey Classification

Uncomplicated diverticulitis: Hinchey 0; complicated: everything else

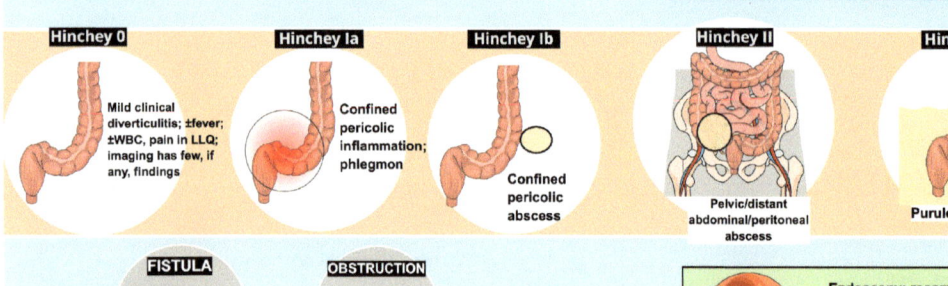

Hinchey 0 — Mild clinical diverticulitis; ±fever; ±WBC, pain in LLQ; imaging has few, if any, findings

Hinchey Ia — Confined pericolic inflammation; phlegmon

Hinchey Ib — Confined pericolic abscess

Hinchey II — Pelvic/distant abdominal/peritoneal abscess

Hinchey III — Purulent peritonitis

Hinchey IV — Fecal peritonitis

FISTULA
colovesical
colenteric
colovaginal
colocutaneous

OBSTRUCTION
colonic ± small bowel

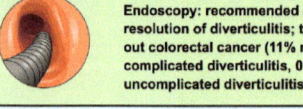

Endoscopy: recommended after resolution of diverticulitis; to rule out colorectal cancer (11% risk with complicated diverticulitis, 0.7% with uncomplicated diverticulitis)

Diverticulitis Treatment

Treatment for diverticulitis is evolving. It may include treatment with or without antibiotics; interventional radiological procedures, minimally invasive or open surgery with or without resection; with or without creation of a stoma

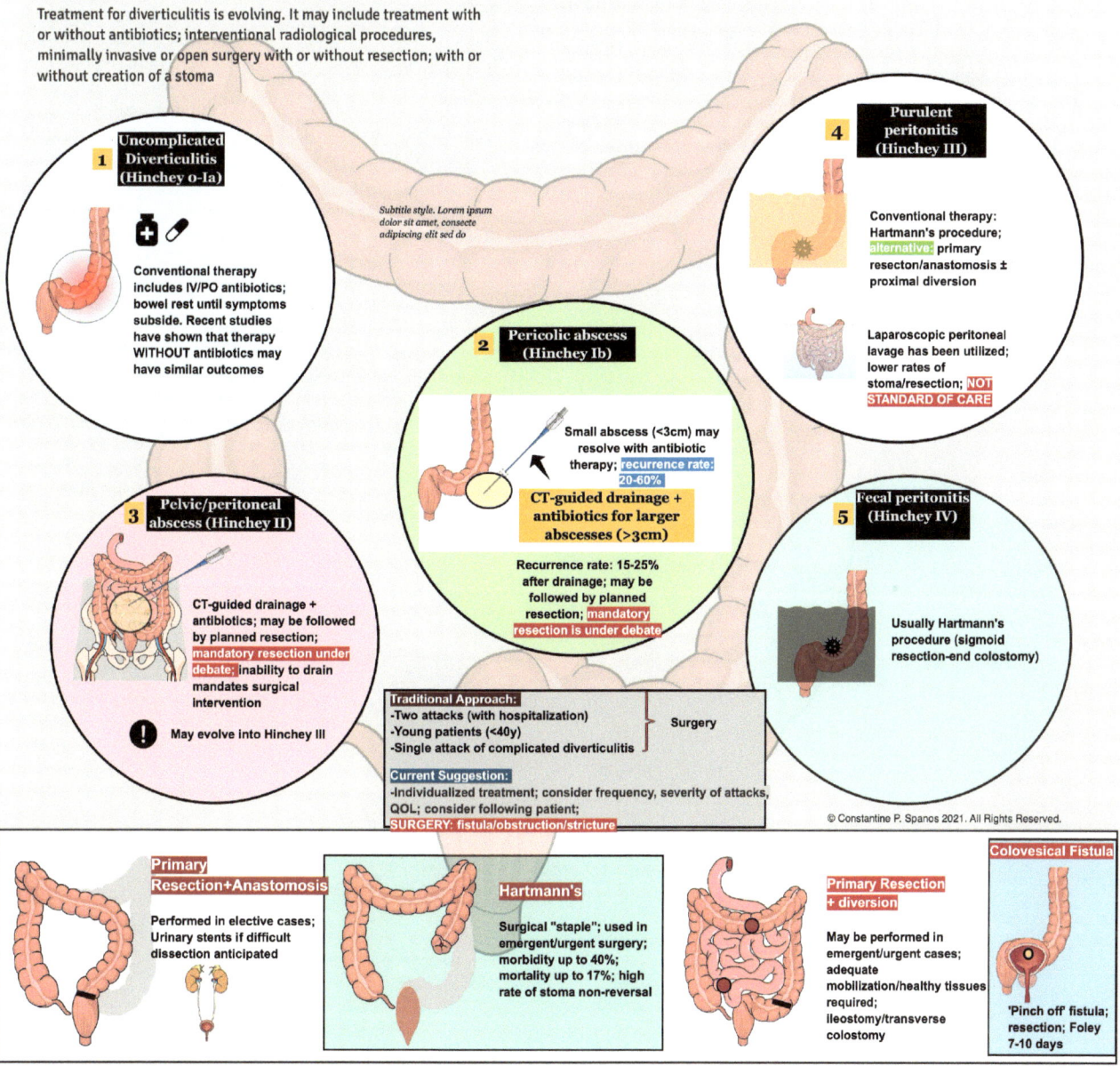

4 Purulent peritonitis (Hinchey III)

Conventional therapy: Hartmann's procedure; alternative: primary resecton/anastomosis ± proximal diversion

Laparoscopic peritoneal lavage has been utilized; lower rates of stoma/resection; NOT STANDARD OF CARE

1 Uncomplicated Diverticulitis (Hinchey 0-Ia)

Conventional therapy includes IV/PO antibiotics; bowel rest until symptoms subside. Recent studies have shown that therapy WITHOUT antibiotics may have similar outcomes

Subtitle style. Lorem ipsum dolor sit amet, consecte adipiscing elit sed do

2 Pericolic abscess (Hinchey Ib)

Small abscess (<3cm) may resolve with antibiotic therapy; recurrence rate: 20-60%

CT-guided drainage + antibiotics for larger abscesses (>3cm)

Recurrence rate: 15-25% after drainage; may be followed by planned resection; mandatory resection is under debate

5 Fecal peritonitis (Hinchey IV)

Usually Hartmann's procedure (sigmoid resection-end colostomy)

3 Pelvic/peritoneal abscess (Hinchey II)

CT-guided drainage + antibiotics; may be followed by planned resection; mandatory resection under debate; inability to drain mandates surgical intervention

May evolve into Hinchey III

Traditional Approach:
-Two attacks (with hospitalization)
-Young patients (<40y)
-Single attack of complicated diverticulitis

Surgery

Current Suggestion:
-Individualized treatment; consider frequency, severity of attacks, QOL; consider following patient;
SURGERY: fistula/obstruction/stricture

Primary Resection+Anastomosis

Performed in elective cases; Urinary stents if difficult dissection anticipated

Hartmann's

Surgical "staple"; used in emergent/urgent surgery; morbidity up to 40%; mortality up to 17%; high rate of stoma non-reversal

Primary Resection + diversion

May be performed in emergent/urgent cases; adequate mobilization/healthy tissues required; ileostomy/transverse colostomy

Colovesical Fistula

'Pinch off' fistula; resection; Foley 7-10 days

Further Reading

Althumairi AA, Gearhart SL. The management of diverticular disease of the colon. In: Cameron JL, Cameron AM, editors. Current surgical therapy. 12th ed. Philadelphia: Elsevier; 2017. p. 149–53.

Diverticular disease of the colon. In: McLatchie G, Borley N, Chikwe J, editors. Oxford handbook of clinical surgery. 4th ed. Oxford: Oxford University Press; 2013. p. 404–5.

Hall J, Hardiman K, Lee S, et al. The American Society of Colon and Rectal Surgeons clinical practice guidelines for the treatment of left-sided colonic diverticulitis. Dis Colon Rectum. 2020;63:728–47.

Mitchem JB, Hunt SR. Colon and rectum. In: Klingensmith ME, Vemuri C, Fayanju OM, Robertson JO, Samson JO, Sanford D, editors. The Washington manual of surgery. 7th ed. Philadelphia: Wolters Kluwer; 2016. p. 422–45.

Schultz JK, Azhar N, Binda JH, et al. European Society of Coloproctology: guidelines for the management of diverticular disease of the colon. Color Dis. 2020; https://doi.org/10.1111/codi.15140.

Silen W. Diverticulitis of the colon. In: Silen W, editor. Cope's early diagnosis of the acute abdomen. 22nd ed. New York: Oxford University Press; 2010. p. 105–7.

- Small bowel obstruction (SBO) is a frequent acute surgical problem. The initial diagnosis is usually straightforward; details regarding etiology, initial and long-term management require diligent clinical assessment and sound judgment.
- The most common etiologies are postoperative adhesions, incarcerated hernias, and malignancies. There are several other etiologies.
- The initial distinction is usually between mechanical bowel obstruction and paralytic ileus.
- Mechanical SBO can be partial or complete. Strangulation is a result of complete SBO usually; vascular compromise of the bowel may lead to infarction and perforation.
- Paralytic ileus occurs when bowel peristalsis is absent. It is a frequent sequela of surgery (postoperative ileus). It can also be caused by electrolyte abnormalities, trauma, peritonitis, systemic infection, uremia, and medications.
- Signs and symptoms of SBO vary according to site and cause of obstruction.
- Pain may be epigastric, periumbilical, and poorly localized. Initially it is colicky (periodic), with peaks and troughs. At the peak of pain, vomiting is common and provides relief.
- With strangulation, the pain becomes steady. If perforation occurs, pain becomes diffuse and severe.
- Vomiting starts earlier in proximal obstruction. Contents are gastric initially, then bilious. Long-standing SBO is characterized by feculent vomiting.
- Obstipation is the absence of flatus and stool; it usually occurs with complete SBO.
- Abdominal distention is more marked with distal SBO.
- Tenderness is increased with distention, strangulation, and perforation. The distinction between localized and diffuse tenderness is very important.
- Patients may be anxious and diaphoretic; they appear quite unwell. Their pulse may be rapid and weak from dehydration. Extremities may be cold, especially in long-standing SBO.
- It is very important to examine all potential hernia orifices (umbilical, inguinal, femoral, and postoperative scars) to rule out incarceration/strangulation. Abdominal incisions in patients with SBO are suggestive of adhesions or cancer recurrence.
- Abdominal auscultation may reveal metallic (high pitched, frequent) sounds initially. Absence of sounds suggests paralytic ileus, strangulation, or perforation.
- The digital rectal exam is important. The presence and quality of contents are revealed; an empty rectal vault is suggestive of complete obstruction.
- Laboratory values may be normal initially. A CBC, electrolyte panel, BUN, creatinine, and glucose are obtained; none are pathognomonic for SBO. Increased WBC, lactate, and amylase in patients with SBO are suggestive of bowel strangulation/necrosis.
- Plain abdominal films (including upright chest) may depict free intraperitoneal air, bowel air-fluid levels, presence or not of gas in colon and rectum. A diagnosis of partial versus complete SBO may be feasible.
- CT scan with triple (PO/IV/Rectal) contrast may determine transition point of obstruction, confirm partial/complete obstruction, and depict intraluminal/extraluminal causes of SBO.
- The differential diagnosis of SBO include pancreatitis, appendicitis, cholecystitis, mesenteric ischemia, renal colic, biliary colic, and ovarian torsion.
- Initial treatment of SBO starts with the assessment of ABCs. Good IV access is obtained; many patients with SBO are volume-depleted; therefore, IV hydration is initiated. Urinary output is monitored (Foley catheter); electrolyte abnormalities are corrected.
- Nasogastric decompression is important. SBO patients are at risk for aspiration.

© The Author(s), under exclusive license to Springer Nature Switzerland AG 2021
C. P. Spanos, *Acute Surgical Topics*, https://doi.org/10.1007/978-3-030-68700-7_9

- Determination of complete versus incomplete SBO is crucial; the goal is to diagnose/prevent strangulation and perforation. Delay in diagnosis may lead to extensive bowel loss, short gut syndrome with associated morbidity/mortality.

- Most cases of incomplete SBO resolve with nonoperative therapy; recurrence is relatively common.
- Indications for surgery include complete SBO, recurrent SBO, strangulation/perforation, and peritonitis. Laparotomy/laparoscopy can be performed.

Bowel Obstruction

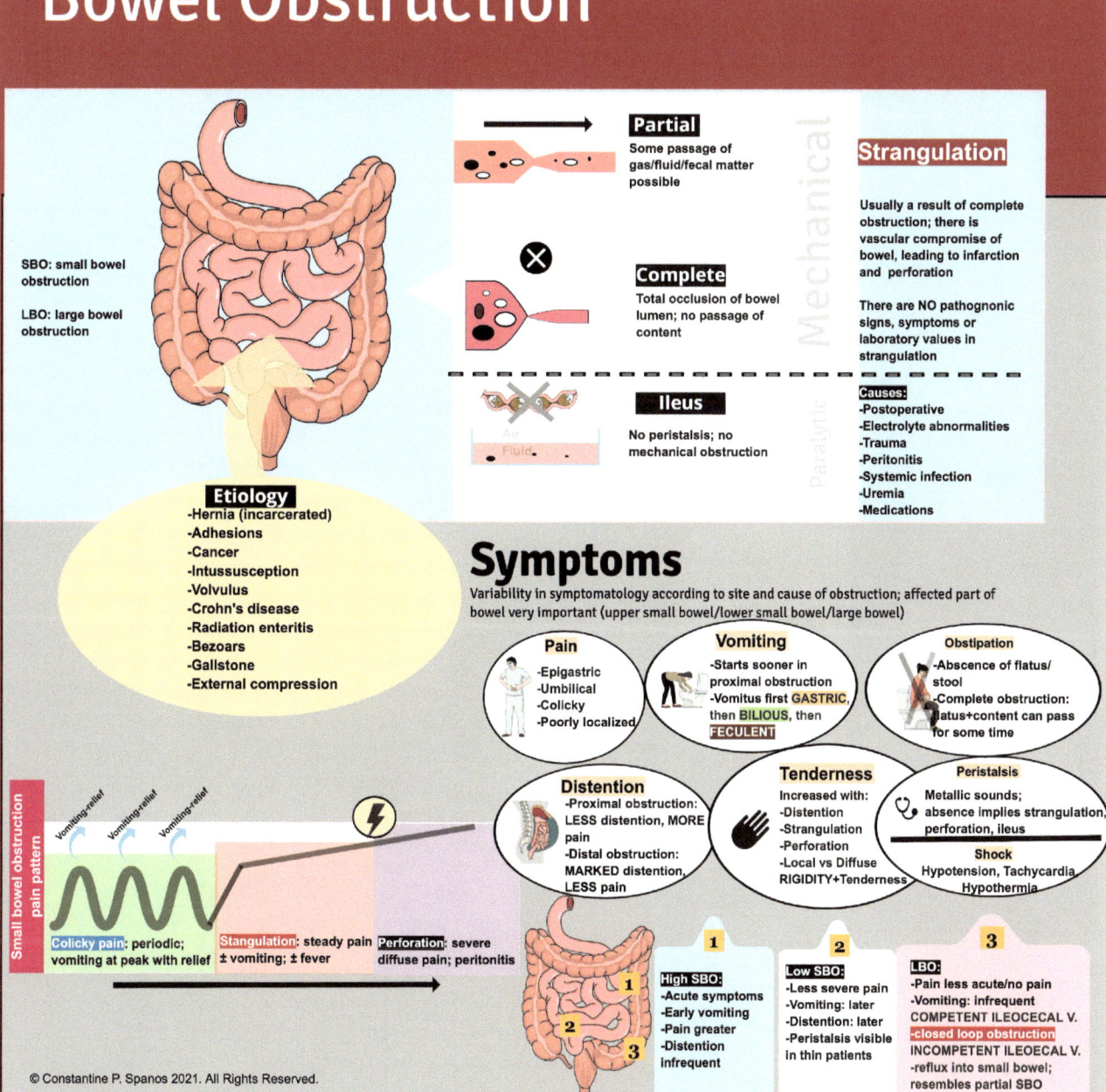

SBO: small bowel obstruction

LBO: large bowel obstruction

Partial
Some passage of gas/fluid/fecal matter possible

Complete
Total occlusion of bowel lumen; no passage of content

Ileus
No peristalsis; no mechanical obstruction

Mechanical

Paralytic

Strangulation

Usually a result of complete obstruction; there is vascular compromise of bowel, leading to infarction and perforation

There are NO pathognomic signs, symptoms or laboratory values in strangulation

Causes:
-Postoperative
-Electrolyte abnormalities
-Trauma
-Peritonitis
-Systemic infection
-Uremia
-Medications

Etiology
-Hernia (incarcerated)
-Adhesions
-Cancer
-Intussusception
-Volvulus
-Crohn's disease
-Radiation enteritis
-Bezoars
-Gallstone
-External compression

Symptoms

Variability in symptomatology according to site and cause of obstruction; affected part of bowel very important (upper small bowel/lower small bowel/large bowel)

Pain
-Epigastric
-Umbilical
-Colicky
-Poorly localized

Vomiting
-Starts sooner in proximal obstruction
-Vomitus first GASTRIC, then BILIOUS, then FECULENT

Obstipation
-Absence of flatus/stool
-Complete obstruction: flatus+content can pass for some time

Distention
-Proximal obstruction: LESS distention, MORE pain
-Distal obstruction: MARKED distention, LESS pain

Tenderness
Increased with:
-Distention
-Strangulation
-Perforation
-Local vs Diffuse RIGIDITY+Tenderness

Peristalsis
Metallic sounds; absence implies strangulation, perforation, ileus

Shock
Hypotension, Tachycardia Hypothermia

Small bowel obstruction pain pattern

Vomiting-relief   Vomiting-relief   Vomiting-relief

Colicky pain: periodic; vomiting at peak with relief

Stangulation: steady pain ± vomiting; ± fever

Perforation: severe diffuse pain; peritonitis

1 High SBO:
-Acute symptoms
-Early vomiting
-Pain greater
-Distention infrequent

2 Low SBO:
-Less severe pain
-Vomiting: later
-Distention: later
-Peristalsis visible in thin patients

3 LBO:
-Pain less acute/no pain
-Vomiting: infrequent
COMPETENT ILEOCECAL V.
-closed loop obstruction
INCOMPETENT ILEOECAL V.
-reflux into small bowel; resembles partial SBO

Small Bowel Obstruction: Evaluation, Treatment

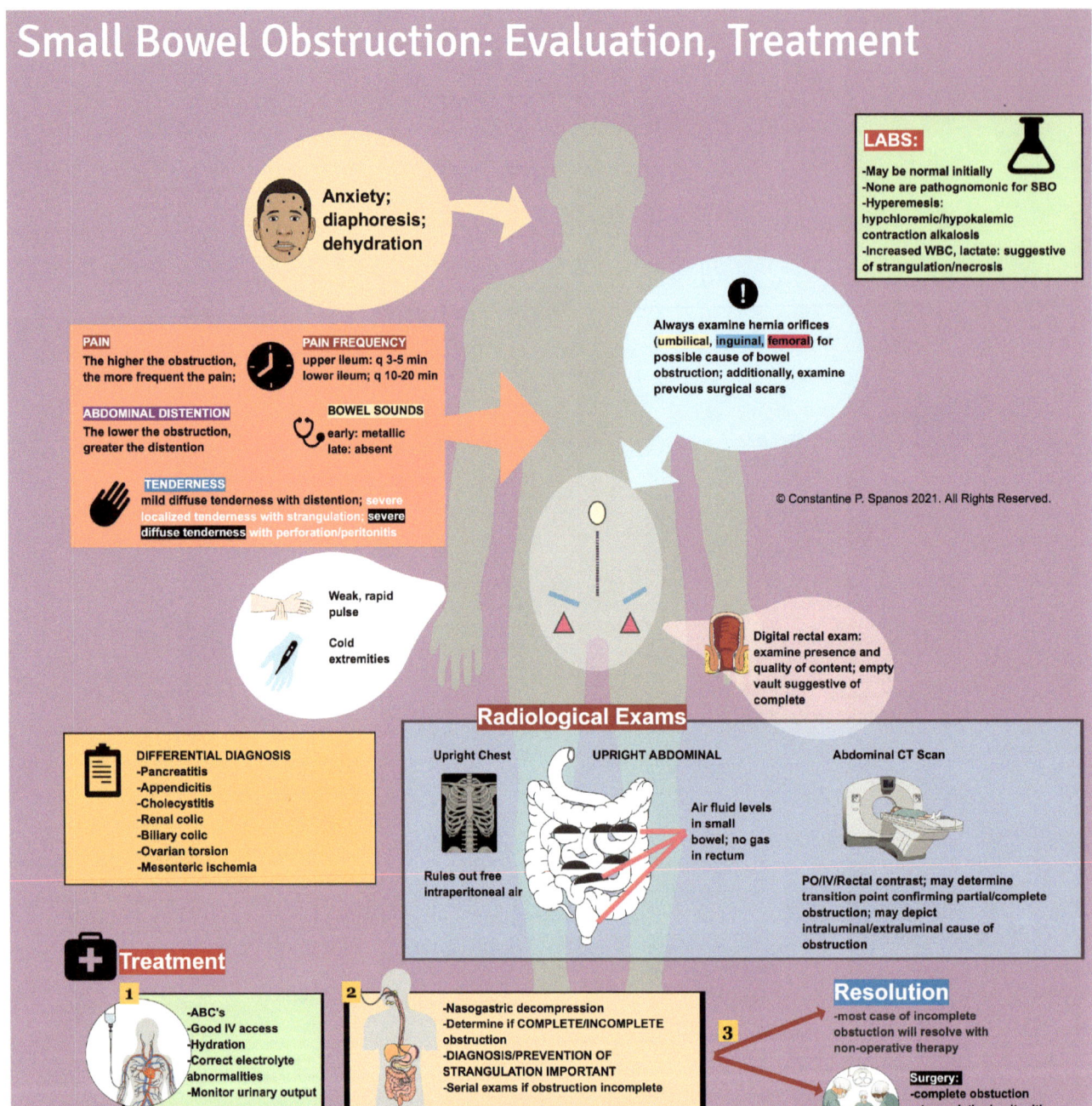

Anxiety; diaphoresis; dehydration

LABS:
-May be normal initially
-None are pathognomonic for SBO
-Hyperemesis: hypchloremic/hypokalemic contraction alkalosis
-Increased WBC, lactate: suggestive of strangulation/necrosis

PAIN
The higher the obstruction, the more frequent the pain;

PAIN FREQUENCY
upper ileum: q 3-5 min
lower ileum; q 10-20 min

ABDOMINAL DISTENTION
The lower the obstruction, greater the distention

BOWEL SOUNDS
early: metallic
late: absent

TENDERNESS
mild diffuse tenderness with distention; severe localized tenderness with strangulation; severe diffuse tenderness with perforation/peritonitis

Always examine hernia orifices (umbilical, inguinal, femoral) for possible cause of bowel obstruction; additionally, examine previous surgical scars

© Constantine P. Spanos 2021. All Rights Reserved.

Weak, rapid pulse

Cold extremities

Digital rectal exam: examine presence and quality of content; empty vault suggestive of complete

DIFFERENTIAL DIAGNOSIS
-Pancreatitis
-Appendicitis
-Cholecystitis
-Renal colic
-Biliary colic
-Ovarian torsion
-Mesenteric ischemia

Radiological Exams

Upright Chest
Rules out free intraperitoneal air

UPRIGHT ABDOMINAL
Air fluid levels in small bowel; no gas in rectum

Abdominal CT Scan
PO/IV/Rectal contrast; may determine transition point confirming partial/complete obstruction; may depict intraluminal/extraluminal cause of obstruction

Treatment

1 -ABC's
-Good IV access
-Hydration
-Correct electrolyte abnormalities
-Monitor urinary output

2 -Nasogastric decompression
-Determine if COMPLETE/INCOMPLETE obstruction
-DIAGNOSIS/PREVENTION OF STRANGULATION IMPORTANT
-Serial exams if obstruction incomplete

3 **Resolution**
-most case of incomplete obstuction will resolve with non-operative therapy

Surgery:
-complete obstuction
-strangulation/peritonitis
-recurrent obstruction

Further Reading

DiBrito SR, Duncan M. The management of small bowel obstruction. In: Cameron JL, Cameron AM, editors. Current surgical therapy. 12th ed. Philadelphia: Elsevier; 2017. p. 109–13.

Leinicke JA, Wise PE. Small intestine. In: Klingensmith ME, Vemuri C, Fayanju OM, Robertson JO, Samson JO, Sanford D, editors. The Washington manual of surgery. 7th ed. Philadelphia: Wolters Kluwer; 2016. p. 339–56.

Silen W. Acute intestinal obstruction. In: Silen W, editor. Cope's early diagnosis of the acute abdomen. 22nd ed. New York: Oxford University Press; 2010. p. 153–77.

- Large bowel obstruction (LBO) differs from SBO in etiology and clinical presentation. A careful history and physical exam often distinguish between the two diagnoses; imaging usually confirms the diagnosis. Left-sided LBO is the most common form.
- LBO is often an indication for emergent/urgent or semiurgent surgery. Initial nonoperative treatment is utilized selectively or palliatively.
- The most common cause of LBO is colorectal cancer (60–80%), followed by diverticular stricture (10–20%) and volvulus (5%). Other causes are Crohn's colitis, radiation colitis, hernia (incarceration of sigmoid colon in a left inguinal hernia), endometriosis, and fecal impaction.
- Colon cancer presents with gradually increasing constipation and change in bowel habits. **Obstipation** is worrisome for complete obstruction. Abdominal distention is initially painless, then associated with cramping as the obstruction progresses. Blood per rectum is frequent; frequently mixed with stool. Patients may be anemic.
- Diverticular stricture may present in a similar fashion. A history of acute diverticulitis is suggestive; colorectal cancer must be ruled out.
- Volvulus presents acutely. There is rapid onset of constipation/obstipation with acute abdominal pain and distention. Colonic vascular compromise in combination with profound colonic distention leads to ischemia, perforation, and peritonitis.
- Vomiting is not as common as in SBO. An LBO with an incompetent ileocecal valve may present similarly to SBO with vomiting.
- Physical exam is notable for significant abdominal distention (greater than in SBO).
- Tenderness is present to a variable degree. A digital rectal exam will rule out a low rectal tumor or fecal impaction.
- Plain abdominal films will depict colonic diameter at various locations. A cecal diameter >12 cm and/or transverse colonic diameter of >6 cm confers a high risk of perforation. A coffee-bean sign is suggestive of sigmoid volvulus. **Air-fluid levels in the small bowel suggest an incompetent ileocecal valve**. A large amount of stool in the rectal area suggests fecal impaction.
- Contrast enemas (water-soluble contrast preferably) are useful to depict the level and morphology of obstruction (e.g., apple-core lesion of colorectal cancer, bird's-beak of sigmoid volvulus) and may be therapeutic in cases of partial LBO and fecal impaction. It is especially useful in the diagnosis of colonic pseudo-obstruction (Ogilvie's).
- CT scan may show site/morphology of lesion, pneumatosis coli, vascular compromise, diameter of colon, extraluminal air or other lesions, metastatic disease in cases of colorectal cancer.
- Endoscopy is used for diagnosis of cancer (with biopsy), stricture or IBD, decompression of volvulus, placement of a stent through cancer, and decompression of colonic pseudo-obstruction.
- Nonoperative treatment for LBO includes enema/disimpaction for fecal impaction, endoscopic detorsion of volvulus ± placement of rectal decompressive tube, reduction of hernia, and stent placement for temporary or palliative alleviation of malignant obstruction.
- Colonic stents can be used as a bridge to resection; they may allow for subsequent colon preparation and total endoscopic evaluation. They may also provide palliation for unresectable lesions or patients unfit for surgery. Complications include migration, colon perforation.
- Emergent/urgent surgical procedures for complete LBO include:
  - Hartmann's procedure
  - Decompressive colostomy prior to point of obstruction; resection later
  - Resection with primary anastomosis ± proximal diversion
  - Resection; on-table colonic lavage; primary anastomosis
  - Subtotal colectomy with ileorectostomy
  - Resection with ileocolostomy for right-sided LBO
  - Hartmann's procedure in cases of perforation and peritonitis

- Initial treatment for sigmoid volvulus is endoscopic detorsion and decompression. Retorsion occurs in 50% of cases; semi-urgent surgery (resection and primary anastomosis) is recommended after successful endoscopic treatment.
- Colonic pseudo-obstruction (Ogilvie's syndrome) is an acute colonic dysmotility syndrome. It is usually encountered in immobilized hospitalized patients with significant coexisting conditions such as severe cardiac disease, spinal fractures, pneumonia, major orthopedic surgery in elderly patients, and hypokalemia. Medications (anticholinergics, anti-depressants, and narcotics) can also cause/exacerbate this condition.

- Patients present with painless distention initially. Tachypnea and tachycardia are common. Tenderness may signal impending perforation.
- Mechanical LBO must be ruled out, CT scan or careful contrast enema may be performed.
- Treatment includes:
  - Correction of metabolic/electrolyte abnormalities
  - Neostigmine (2 mg over 10–20 min IV) with cardiac monitoring. This may lead to bradycardia, which can be reversed with atropine.
  - Colonoscopic decompression.
  - Surgery is indicated when other options fail, or when perforation occurs. It is associated with significant morbidity and mortality.

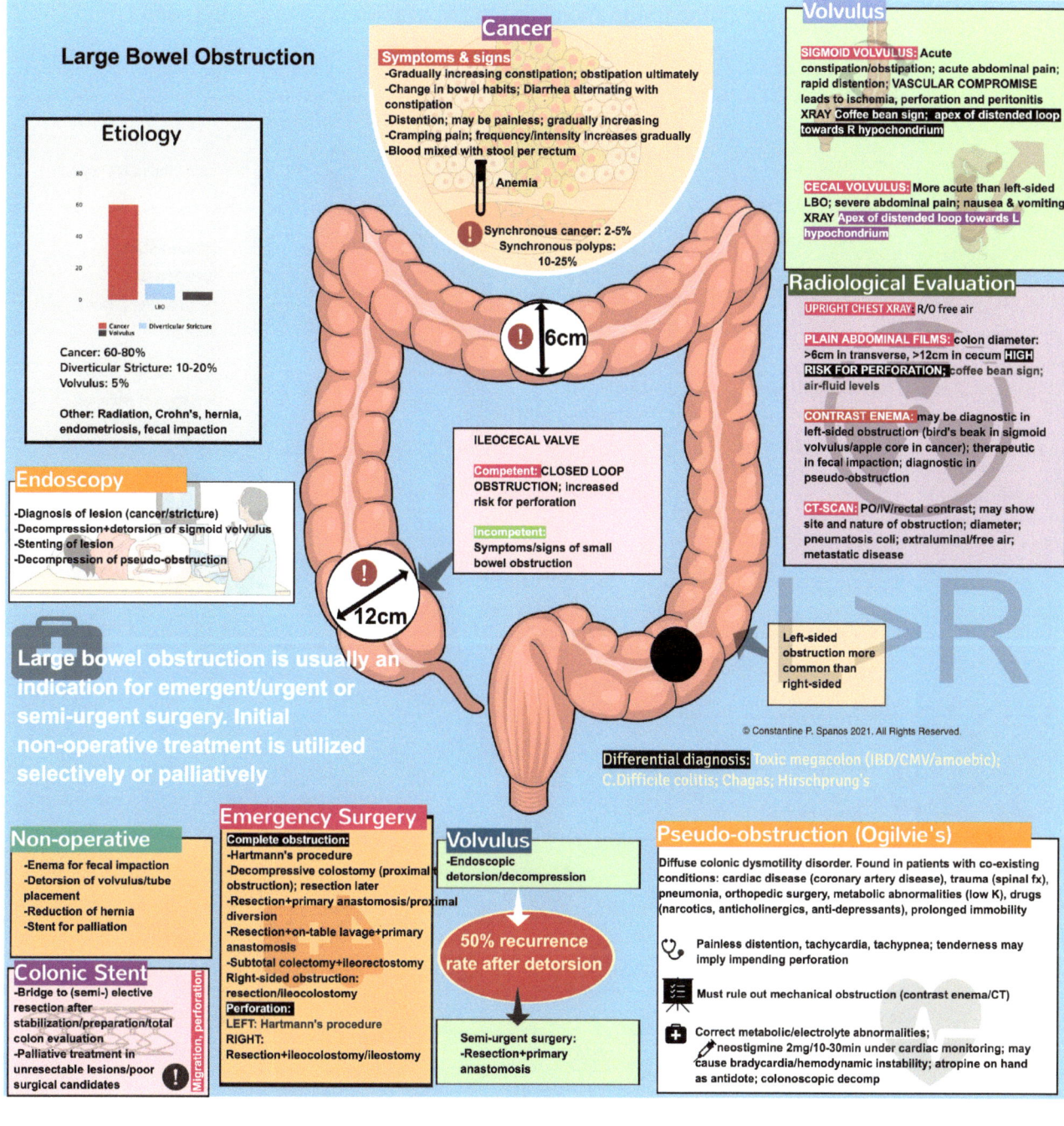

Large Bowel Obstruction

Etiology

Cancer: 60-80%
Diverticular Stricture: 10-20%
Volvulus: 5%

Other: Radiation, Crohn's, hernia, endometriosis, fecal impaction

Cancer

Symptoms & signs
-Gradually increasing constipation; obstipation ultimately
-Change in bowel habits; Diarrhea alternating with constipation
-Distention; may be painless; gradually increasing
-Cramping pain; frequency/intensity increases gradually
-Blood mixed with stool per rectum

Anemia

Synchronous cancer: 2-5%
Synchronous polyps: 10-25%

Volvulus

SIGMOID VOLVULUS: Acute constipation/obstipation; acute abdominal pain; rapid distention; VASCULAR COMPROMISE leads to ischemia, perforation and peritonitis XRAY Coffee bean sign; apex of distended loop towards R hypochondrium

CECAL VOLVULUS: More acute than left-sided LBO; severe abdominal pain; nausea & vomiting XRAY Apex of distended loop towards L hypochondrium

Radiological Evaluation

UPRIGHT CHEST XRAY: R/O free air

PLAIN ABDOMINAL FILMS: colon diameter: >6cm in transverse, >12cm in cecum HIGH RISK FOR PERFORATION; coffee bean sign; air-fluid levels

CONTRAST ENEMA: may be diagnostic in left-sided obstruction (bird's beak in sigmoid volvulus/apple core in cancer); therapeutic in fecal impaction; diagnostic in pseudo-obstruction

CT-SCAN: PO/IV/rectal contrast; may show site and nature of obstruction; diameter; pneumatosis coli; extraluminal/free air; metastatic disease

Endoscopy

-Diagnosis of lesion (cancer/stricture)
-Decompression+detorsion of sigmoid volvulus
-Stenting of lesion
-Decompression of pseudo-obstruction

6cm

12cm

ILEOCECAL VALVE

Competent: CLOSED LOOP OBSTRUCTION; increased risk for perforation

Incompetent: Symptoms/signs of small bowel obstruction

Left-sided obstruction more common than right-sided

L > R

Large bowel obstruction is usually an indication for emergent/urgent or semi-urgent surgery. Initial non-operative treatment is utilized selectively or palliatively

Differential diagnosis: Toxic megacolon (IBD/CMV/amoebic); C.Difficile colitis; Chagas; Hirschprung's

Non-operative

-Enema for fecal impaction
-Detorsion of volvulus/tube placement
-Reduction of hernia
-Stent for palliation

Colonic Stent

-Bridge to (semi-) elective resection after stabilization/preparation/total colon evaluation
-Palliative treatment in unresectable lesions/poor surgical candidates

Migration, perforation

Emergency Surgery

Complete obstruction:
-Hartmann's procedure
-Decompressive colostomy (proximal obstruction); resection later
-Resection+primary anastomosis/proximal diversion
-Resection+on-table lavage+primary anastomosis
-Subtotal colectomy+ileorectostomy
Right-sided obstruction: resection/ileocolostomy
Perforation:
LEFT: Hartmann's procedure
RIGHT: Resection+ileocolostomy/ileostomy

Volvulus

-Endoscopic detorsion/decompression

50% recurrence rate after detorsion

Semi-urgent surgery:
-Resection+primary anastomosis

Pseudo-obstruction (Ogilvie's)

Diffuse colonic dysmotility disorder. Found in patients with co-existing conditions: cardiac disease (coronary artery disease), trauma (spinal fx), pneumonia, orthopedic surgery, metabolic abnormalities (low K), drugs (narcotics, anticholinergics, anti-depressants), prolonged immobility

Painless distention, tachycardia, tachypnea; tenderness may imply impending perforation

Must rule out mechanical obstruction (contrast enema/CT)

Correct metabolic/electrolyte abnormalities; neostigmine 2mg/10-30min under cardiac monitoring; may cause bradycardia/hemodynamic instability; atropine on hand as antidote; colonoscopic decomp

Clostridiodes difficile infection

Clinical Manifestations

Asymptomatic carrier: No signs or symptoms

Mild: Mild diarrhea, afebrile, mild abdominal pain/tenderness, labs mostly normal

Moderate: Moderate non-bloody diarrhea, moderate abdominal pain/tenderness, nausea/vomiting, dehydration, WBC>15,000, BUN/creatinine above normal

Severe: Severe ±bloody diarrhea, pseudomembranous colitis, severe abdominal pain/tenderness, vomiting, ileus, T>38.9C, WBC>20,000; albumin <2.5 mg/dl, acute kidney injury

Fulminant: Toxic megacolon, peritonitis, respiratory distress, hemodynamic instability

Endoscopy

-Pseudomembranes pathognomonic
-Useful in patients with IBD
-Full colonoscopy is preferred; right-sided colitis in 30%
-Fulminant colitis is a contraindication

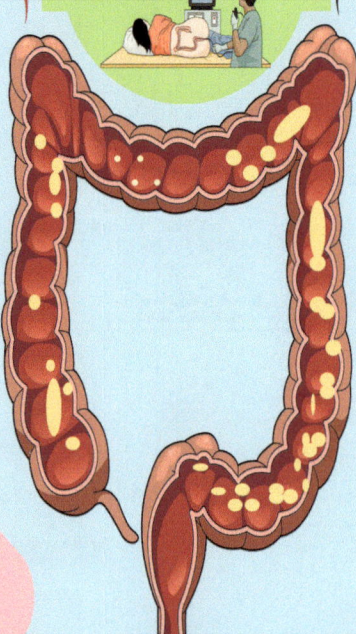

Prevention

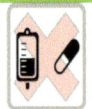

Minimize antibiotic usage

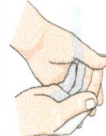

Handwashing (soap+water) before/after patient contact

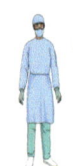

Isolation of patients diagnosed with C. difficile infection; healthcare providers don gown+gloves

Probiotics: mixed results

Diagnosis

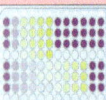

Enzyme immunoassay: detects toxin A, B in stool

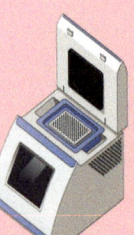

DNA-based tests (PCR): identify microbial toxin genes in stool; most accurate (95% negative predictive value)

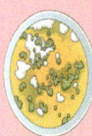

Stool culture: not widely available

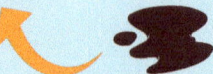

Diarrhea is a prerequisite for testing-solid stool is not an indication for testing

Treatment: C. difficile colitis

VANCOMYCIN, METRONIDAZOLE; mainstay of treatment

Asymptomatic carrier: NO TREATMENT

Mild: Stop predisposing antibiotics; hydration; METRONIDAZOLE 500mg PO TID for 10-14 days

Moderate: Stop predisposing antibiotics; hydration; METRONIDAZOLE 500mg PO TID or VANCOMYCIN 125mg PO QID for 10-14 days

Severe: Hydration; close clinical monitoring; VANCOMYCIN (PO/per NG/retention enema) 500mg QID ± METRONIDAZOLE 500mg IV TID; if risk of recurrence high: FIDAXOMYCIN 200mg PO BID for 10 days

Fulminant: Antibiotics as for severe colitis; surgical consultation

INDICATIONS FOR SURGERY
-Peritonitis
-Perforation
-Severe, fulminant colitis not improving after 12-24h of medical therapy

Surgical Procedures

-Subtotal colectomy + end ileostomy
-Diverting ileostomy, colonic lavage; postoperative antegrade colonic irrigation with VANCOMYCIN through stoma

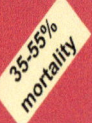

35-55% mortality

FIDAXOMYCIN

Novel, poorly absorbed, bactericidal, macrocyclic activity against anaerobic Gram + bacteria
15% recurrent colitis vs 25% for vancomycin

$$$$

Other antibiotics
Rifaximin, teicoplanin, tigecycline, ramoplanin; NOT USUALLY RECOMMENDED

Fecal Microbial Transplantation

Fecal material from healthy, tested donor(s) administered to patient orally or rectally; Bacteriodetes/Firmicutes phylla critical components

Vaccine

Vaccine trials underway to induce IgG antitoxin production

Recurrent Infection (up to 30%)

FIRST RECURRENCE: VANCOMYCIN 125mg PO QID or METRONIDAZOLE 500mg PO TID for 10-14 days

SECOND RECURRENCE: FIDAXOMYCIN 200mg PO BID for 10 days; consider fecal microbial transplantation

Further Reading

Alavi K, Friel CM. Large bowel obstruction. In: Steele SR, Hull TR, Read TE, Saclarides TJ, Senagore AJ, Whitlow CB, editors. The ASCRS textbook of colon and rectal surgery. 3rd ed. Heidelberg: Springer; 2016. p. 669–96.

Fabrizio AC, Wick EC. The management of large bowel obstruction. In: Cameron JL, Cameron AM, editors. Current surgical therapy. 12th ed. Philadelphia: Elsevier; 2017. p. 180–2.

Mitchem JB, Hunt SR. Colon and rectum. In: Klingensmith ME, Vemuri C, Fayanju OM, Robertson JO, Samson JO, Sanford D, editors. The Washington manual of surgery. 7th ed. Philadelphia: Wolters Kluwer; 2016. p. 422–45.

Silen W. Acute intestinal obstruction. In: Silen W, editor. Cope's early diagnosis of the acute abdomen. 22nd ed. New York: Oxford University Press; 2010. p. 153–77.

- *Clostridioides difficile* (*C. diff*) is the most frequently reported nosocomial pathogen and a leading cause of morbidity and mortality in hospitalized patients. In the USA 435,000 infections are annually reported, with 29,000 deaths. *C. diff* infection quadruples hospitalization costs.
- *Clostridioides difficile* is an anaerobic, Gram-positive, spore-forming toxin-producing bacillus. It resides within the gut flora. In health, *C. diff* colonization is prevented by the barrier properties of fecal microbiota in the colon. Antibiotic usage diminishes fecal microbiota, leading to colonic colonization with toxigenic *C. diff*. The toxins released by *C. diff* cause colonocyte death and neutrophilic colitis.
- Risk factors for *C. diff* colitis include antibiotic usage, advanced age, hospitalization, inflammatory bowel disease, organ transplantation, immunosuppression, chemotherapy, and chronic renal failure.
- Use of any type of antibiotic may be associated with the development of *C. diff* colitis. Currently, the most common culprits are ampicillin, amoxicillin, cephalosporins, clindamycin, and fluoroquinolones.
- Of note, a more virulent strain of *C. diff* has been reported: B1/NAP1/027. It is characterized by more efficient sporulation and toxin production and a higher mortality rate. Fluoroquinolone resistance is higher as well.
- The hospital environment is contaminated by spores shed in patients' stool. When infectious precautions are lacking, hospital personnel may infect other patients.
- The most effective preventative measure is handwashing with soap and water by hospital personnel and patients. Alcohol-based sanitizers are not as effective.
- *C. diff* colitis severity can be classified as follows:
  - Asymptomatic carrier, with no signs or symptoms.
  - Mild colitis; mild diarrhea and abdominal pain/tenderness, without fever.
  - Moderate colitis; moderate non-bloody diarrhea, abdominal pain and tenderness, nausea/vomiting, WBC > 15,000, abnormal BUN/creatinine.
  - Severe colitis; severe diarrhea, which may be bloody. Severe abdominal pain/microbial toxin genes in stool and are the most accurate. Stool cultures are not widely available. Tenderness, vomiting, fever >38.9 °C, WBC > 20,000, hypoalbuminemia, and acute kidney injury.
  - Fulminant colitis; Toxic megacolon, peritonitis, respiratory distress, and hemodynamic instability.
- Laboratory diagnosis is based on sampling the patient's stool. Diarrhea is a prerequisite. Enzyme immunoassays detect toxin A, B in stool. DNA-based tests (PCR) identify microbial toxin genes in stool and are the most accurate. Stool cultures for *C. diff* are not widely available.
- Endoscopy confirms the presence of pseudomembranes, which are pathognomonic. It is useful in IBD patients since right-sided colitis is present in a third of patients. Endoscopy should not be performed in patients with severe/fulminant colitis, as there is an increased risk of perforation.
- Treatment depends on disease severity. The mainstay of treatment includes enteral vancomycin or enteral metronidazole in most cases of mild/moderate colitis. Enteral vancomycin ± parenteral metronidazole is used in severe/fulminant colitis. Enteral fidaxomycin can be used in severe/fulminant colitis.
- Surgical consultation is obtained in severe/fulminant colitis. Indications for surgery include severe/fulminant colitis not improving after 12–24 h of medical therapy, peritonitis, and perforation.
- Surgical procedures performed for severe/fulminant colitis include subtotal colectomy with end ileostomy, and diverting ileostomy, colonic lavage with postoperative antegrade colonic irrigation with vancomycin through stoma. Surgery has a 35–55% mortality rate.
- Fecal microbial transplantation is a novel modality in which fecal material from healthy donors is administered to patients orally or rectally.
- Vaccine trials to induce IgG antitoxin production are currently underway.

C. P. Spanos, *Acute Surgical Topics*, https://doi.org/10.1007/978-3-030-68700-7_11

- Recurrent *C. diff* infection occurs in 30% of patients. The use of fidaxomicin is known to reduce recurrence rates.
- Prevention of *C. diff* development and nosocomial spread is key. This is achieved primarily by minimizing antibiotic use. Soap and water handwashing before and after patient contact, isolation of infected patients, and preventive protective equipment (gown and gloves) for personnel are paramount. Probiotic administration has shown mixed results.

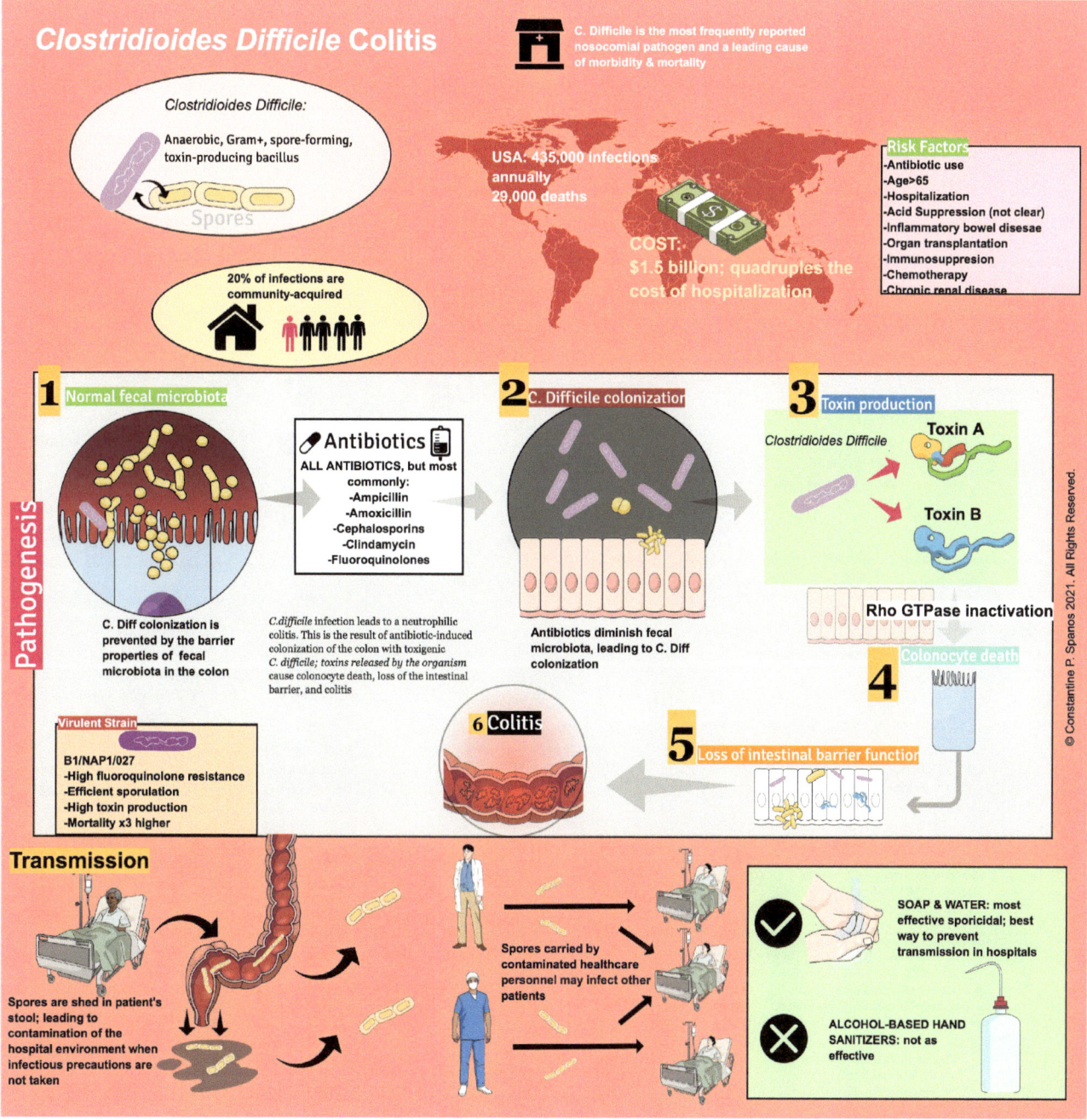

Clostridioides Difficile Colitis

C. Difficile is the most frequently reported nosocomial pathogen and a leading cause of morbidity & mortality

Clostridioides Difficile:
Anaerobic, Gram+, spore-forming, toxin-producing bacillus

Spores

USA: 435,000 infections annually
29,000 deaths

COST: $1.5 billion; quadruples the cost of hospitalization

20% of infections are community-acquired

Risk Factors
-Antibiotic use
-Age>65
-Hospitalization
-Acid Suppression (not clear)
-Inflammatory bowel disesae
-Organ transplantation
-Immunosuppresion
-Chemotherapy
-Chronic renal disease

Pathogenesis

1 Normal fecal microbiota

C. Diff colonization is prevented by the barrier properties of fecal microbiota in the colon

Antibiotics
ALL ANTIBIOTICS, but most commonly:
-Ampicillin
-Amoxicillin
-Cephalosporins
-Clindamycin
-Fluoroquinolones

C.difficile infection leads to a neutrophilic colitis. This is the result of antibiotic-induced colonization of the colon with toxigenic *C. difficile*; toxins released by the organism cause colonocyte death, loss of the intestinal barrier, and colitis

2 C. Difficile colonization

Antibiotics diminish fecal microbiota, leading to C. Diff colonization

3 Toxin production

Clostridioides Difficile

Toxin A

Toxin B

Rho GTPase inactivation

4 Colonocyte death

5 Loss of intestinal barrier function

6 Colitis

Virulent Strain
B1/NAP1/027
-High fluoroquinolone resistance
-Efficient sporulation
-High toxin production
-Mortality x3 higher

Transmission

Spores are shed in patient's stool; leading to contamination of the hospital environment when infectious precautions are not taken

Spores carried by contaminated healthcare personnel may infect other patients

✓ SOAP & WATER: most effective sporicidal; best way to prevent transmission in hospitals

✗ ALCOHOL-BASED HAND SANITIZERS: not as effective

Clostridiodes difficile infection

Clinical Manifestations

Asymptomatic carrier: No signs or symptoms

Mild: Mild diarrhea, afebrile, mild abdominal pain/tenderness, labs mostly normal

Moderate: Moderate non-bloody diarrhea, moderate abdominal pain/tenderness, nausea/vomiting, dehydration, WBC>15,000, BUN/creatinine above normal

Severe: Severe ±bloody diarrhea, pseudomembranous colitis, severe abdominal pain/tenderness, vomiting, ileus, T>38.9C, WBC>20,000; albumin <2.5 mg/dl, acute kidney injury

Fulminant: Toxic megacolon, peritonitis, respiratory distress, hemodynamic instability

Diagnosis

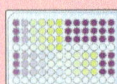

Enzyme immunoassay: detects toxin A, B in stool

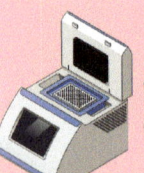

DNA-based tests (PCR): identify microbial toxin genes in stool; most accurate (95% negative predictive value)

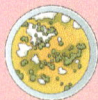

Stool culture: not widely available

FIDAXOMYCIN

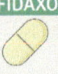

Novel, poorly absorbed, bactericidal, macrocyclic activity against anaerobic Gram + bacteria
15% recurrent colitis vs 25% for vancomycin

Fecal Microbial Transplantation

Fecal material from healthy, tested donor(s) administered to patient orally or rectally; Bacteriodetes/Firmicutes phyla critical components

Vaccine

Vaccine trials underway to induce IgG antitoxin production

Endoscopy

-Pseudomembranes pathognomonic
-Useful in patients with IBD
-Full colonoscopy is preferred; right-sided colitis in 30%
-Fulminant colitis is a contraindication

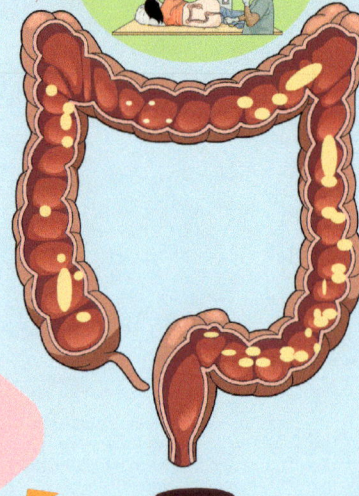

Diarrhea is a prerequisite for testing-solid stool is not an indication for testing

Other antibiotics

Rifaximin, teicoplanin, tigecycline, ramoplanin; NOT USUALLY RECOMMENDED

Recurrent Infection (up to 30%)

FIRST RECURRENCE: VANCOMYCIN 125mg PO QID or METRONIDAZOLE 500mg PO TID for 10-14 days

SECOND RECURRENCE: FIDAXOMYCIN 200mg PO BID for 10 days; consider fecal microbial transplantation

Prevention

Minimize antibiotic usage

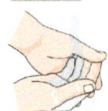

Handwashing (soap+water) before/after patient contact

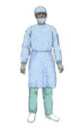

Isolation of patients diagnosed with C. difficile infection; healthcare providers don gown+gloves

Probiotics: mixed results

Treatment: C. difficile colitis

VANCOMYCIN, METRONIDAZOLE; mainstay of treatment

Asymptomatic carrier: NO TREATMENT

Mild: Stop predisposing antibiotics; hydration; METRONIDAZOLE 500mg PO TID for 10-14 days

Moderate: Stop predisposing antibiotics; hydration; METRONIDAZOLE 500mg PO TID or VANCOMYCIN 125mg PO QID for 10-14 days

Severe: Hydration; close clinical monitoring; VANCOMYCIN (PO/per NG/retention enema) 500mg QID ± METRONIDAZOLE 500mg IV TID; if risk of recurrence high: FIDAXOMYCIN 200mg PO BID for 10 days

Fulminant: Antibiotics as for severe colitis; surgical consultation

INDICATIONS FOR SURGERY

-Peritonitis
-Perforation
-Severe, fulminant colitis not improving after 12-24h of medical therapy

Surgical Procedures

-Subtotal colectomy + end ileostomy
-Diverting ileostomy, colonic lavage; postoperative antegrade colonic irrigation with VANCOMYCIN through stoma

35-55% mortality

Further Reading

Leffler DA, Lamont JT. Clostridium difficile infection. N Engl J Med. 2015;372:1539–48.

Stanley JD, Dart BW IV. The management of Clostridium difficile colitis. In: Cameron JL, Cameron AM, editors. Current surgical therapy. 12th ed. Philadelphia: Elsevier; 2017. p. 176–9.

- Upper gastrointestinal bleeding is defined as bleeding proximal to the ligament of Treitz. The diagnosis is easier to make than for LGIB; etiologies are fewer and treatment is frequently successful with nonoperative treatment. Following are several frequent causes of UGIB.
- Peptic ulcer disease is the most common cause of UGIB. *Helicobacter pylori* is etiopathogenic. Risk factors for peptic ulcer disease include medications (aspirin/NSAIDS), alcohol consumption, and smoking. Patients may have a chronic history of abdominal pain, suggestive of the diagnosis.
- A Mallory-Weiss tear may occur after a bout of excessive vomiting and retching. The tear occurs at the gastroesophageal junction.
- Esophageal varices may cause massive UGIB. A key point in the history would be alcohol abuse, cirrhosis, and hepatic failure.
- Gastric cancer is associated with anorexia, weight loss, and cachexia; patient may also have anemia from chronic blood loss.
- Marginal ulcers develop after gastrointestinal anastomoses constructed in gastrectomy or a gastric bypass procedure for obesity. UGIB of variable severity may occur.
- An aortoduodenal fistula develops after open repair of an abdominal aortic aneurysm and may cause massive UGIB.
- UGIB manifests clinically as hematemesis, coffee-ground emesis, melena, or hematochezia.
- Patients' use of "risky drugs" is extremely important in history-taking:
  - Ulcerogenic drugs: NSAIDs/COX-2 inhibitors
  - Bleeding promoters: aspirin/clopidogrel/anticoagulants
  - Other associated drugs: SSRI/Ca++ channel blockers/aldosterone antagonists
  - Iron/bismuth may turn stool black (melena "false positive")
- The initial management of UGIB starts with the assessment of the patient's hemodynamic status. Massive UGIB may manifest with orthostatic or profound hypotension, tachycardia, chest pain, and shortness of breath. **Remember your ABC's!**
- Intubation may be necessary in massive UGIB, agitation, and respiratory distress and patients at great risk for aspiration.
- Two antecubital, large bore (14–16 gauge) IV cannula provide optimal access for fluid resuscitation and blood/component transfusion. A Foley catheter is placed, and noninvasive hemodynamic monitoring is initiated immediately.
- A NG tube is placed for diagnosis, prevention of aspiration, and lavage for endoscopy preparation. Bilious material effectively rules out upper GI bleeding. Return of blood/bloody material reveals an upper GI source. **Return of clear fluid cannot rule out upper GI bleeding.**
- A CBC, PT/PTT, blood type, and crossmatch are immediately obtained. Transfusion of O negative blood may be necessary when type-matched blood is unavailable.
- Initial resuscitation includes a crystalloid fluid bolus (0.5–1 lt) with frequent or continuous blood pressure monitoring to assess response. Transfusion thresholds are a Hb <7 mg/dl for younger patients, 9 mg/dl for older patients.
- INR is checked to assess coagulopathy. Component transfusion is initiated when INR >2.5. For every 4 units of PRBC, 1 unit of FFP should be transfused.
- Hypovolemia may be assessed by clinical signs. Tachycardia suggests moderate hypovolemia. Orthostatic hypotension suggests a blood volume loss of <15%. Supine hypotension suggests a blood volume loss of >40%
- On physical exam one should carefully look for abdominal scars, assess for pain/tenderness/distension as well as signs of hepatic disease (hepatomegaly, splenomegaly, palmar erythema, caput medusa).
- Upper endoscopy is the cornerstone of UGIB diagnosis and treatment. Nasogastric lavage with room-temperature water facilitates dissolution and aspiration of blood clots,

which may impede endoscopy. Erythromycin is given to facilitate gastric peristalsis and content propulsion.

- Endoscopy should be performed within 12–24 h of UGIB. The **Forrest classification** describes endoscopic findings related to bleeding risk:
    - Ia: active spurting bleeder
    - Ib: oozing
    - IIa: visible non-bleeding vessel
    - IIb: adherent clot
    - IIc: flat-pigment spot
    - III: clear ulcer base
- Hemostasis can be achieved with heater probes, ethanol or epinephrine injection, clips, monopolar/bipolar diathermy, or argon plasma.
- Adjunctive medications include infusion of IV PPI (esomeprazole 80 mg bolus, then 40 mg IV q 12 h). If hemostasis is achieved, esomeprazole is continued for 72 h (decreased rebleeding rates).

- Long-term treatment consists of *Helicobacter pylori* eradication, sucralfate, antacids, H2-blockers.
- Selective angiography can be performed either by infusion of a vasoconstricting agent (e.g., vasopressin) or embolization with coils, gelfoam, or PVC. Vasopressin is reserved for bleeding esophageal varices; it is ineffective in bleeding duodenal ulcers, which are secondary to gastroduodenal artery hemorrhage, a relatively large vessel.
- Indications for surgical treatment include failure to identify or control ongoing bleeding endoscopically combined with massive (>6 U PRBC) transfusion, and when angiography is not available. Duodenotomy, suture-ligature of bleeding vessel, pyloroplasty, and vagotomy are performed for bleeding duodenal ulcer. Vagotomy + antrectomy/ulcer excision is performed for a bleeding gastric ulcer.

Upper Gastrointestinal Bleeding

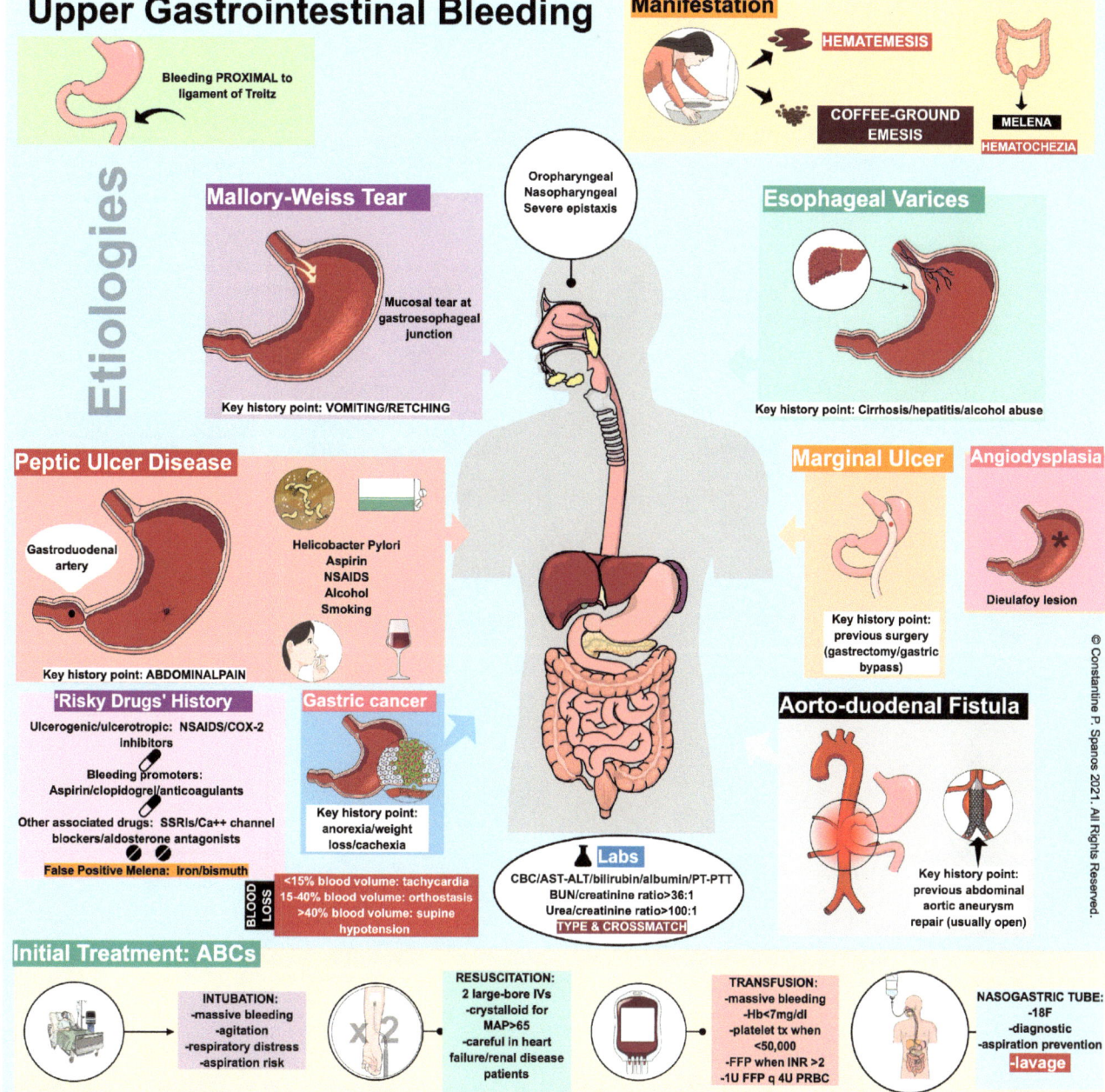

Bleeding PROXIMAL to ligament of Treitz

Etiologies

Manifestation
HEMATEMESIS
COFFEE-GROUND EMESIS
MELENA
HEMATOCHEZIA

Mallory-Weiss Tear
Mucosal tear at gastroesophageal junction

Key history point: VOMITING/RETCHING

Oropharyngeal
Nasopharyngeal
Severe epistaxis

Esophageal Varices
Key history point: Cirrhosis/hepatitis/alcohol abuse

Peptic Ulcer Disease
Gastroduodenal artery

Helicobacter Pylori
Aspirin
NSAIDS
Alcohol
Smoking

Key history point: ABDOMINALPAIN

Marginal Ulcer
Key history point: previous surgery (gastrectomy/gastric bypass)

Angiodysplasia
Dieulafoy lesion

'Risky Drugs' History
Ulcerogenic/ulcerotropic: NSAIDS/COX-2 inhibitors

Bleeding promoters: Aspirin/clopidogrel/anticoagulants

Other associated drugs: SSRIs/Ca++ channel blockers/aldosterone antagonists

False Positive Melena: Iron/bismuth

Gastric cancer
Key history point: anorexia/weight loss/cachexia

BLOOD LOSS
<15% blood volume: tachycardia
15-40% blood volume: orthostasis
>40% blood volume: supine hypotension

Aorto-duodenal Fistula
Key history point: previous abdominal aortic aneurysm repair (usually open)

Labs
CBC/AST-ALT/bilirubin/albumin/PT-PTT
BUN/creatinine ratio>36:1
Urea/creatinine ratio>100:1
TYPE & CROSSMATCH

Initial Treatment: ABCs

INTUBATION:
-massive bleeding
-agitation
-respiratory distress
-aspiration risk

RESUSCITATION:
2 large-bore IVs
-crystalloid for MAP>65
-careful in heart failure/renal disease patients

TRANSFUSION:
-massive bleeding
-Hb<7mg/dl
-platelet tx when <50,000
-FFP when INR >2
-1U FFP q 4U PRBC

NASOGASTRIC TUBE:
-18F
-diagnostic
-aspiration prevention
-lavage

Upper Gastrointestinal Bleeding

Treatment

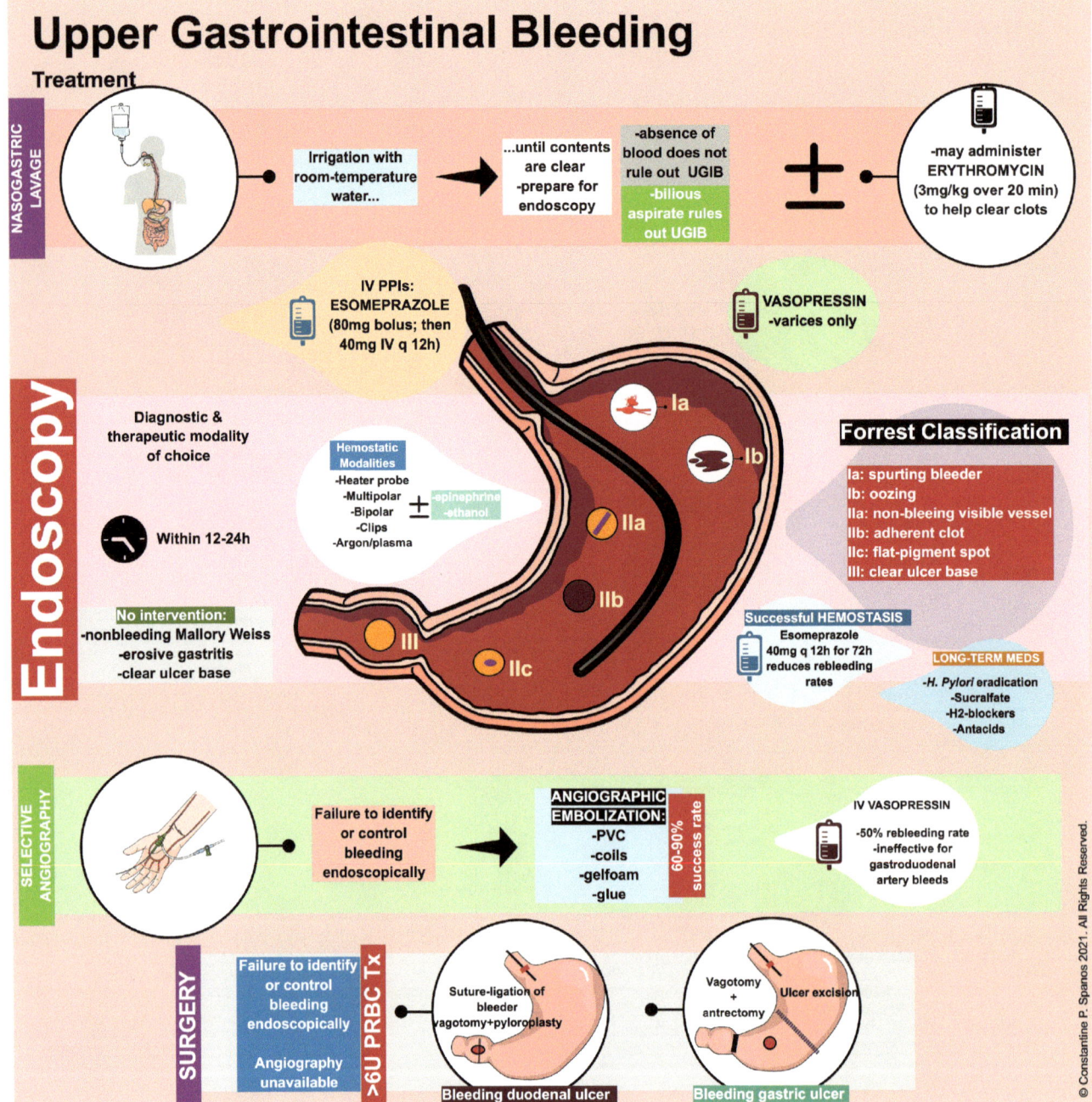

NASOGASTRIC LAVAGE

Irrigation with room-temperature water...

...until contents are clear
-prepare for endoscopy

-absence of blood does not rule out UGIB
-bilious aspirate rules out UGIB

±

-may administer ERYTHROMYCIN (3mg/kg over 20 min) to help clear clots

IV PPIs:
ESOMEPRAZOLE
(80mg bolus; then 40mg IV q 12h)

VASOPRESSIN
-varices only

Endoscopy

Diagnostic & therapeutic modality of choice

Within 12-24h

Hemostatic Modalities
-Heater probe
-Multipolar
-Bipolar
-Clips
-Argon/plasma
± -epinephrine -ethanol

No intervention:
-nonbleeding Mallory Weiss
-erosive gastritis
-clear ulcer base

Ia
Ib
IIa
IIb
III
IIc

Forrest Classification

Ia: spurting bleeder
Ib: oozing
IIa: non-bleeing visible vessel
IIb: adherent clot
IIc: flat-pigment spot
III: clear ulcer base

Successful HEMOSTASIS
Esomeprazole 40mg q 12h for 72h reduces rebleeding rates

LONG-TERM MEDS
-*H. Pylori* eradication
-Sucralfate
-H2-blockers
-Antacids

SELECTIVE ANGIOGRAPHY

Failure to identify or control bleeding endoscopically

ANGIOGRAPHIC EMBOLIZATION:
-PVC
-coils
-gelfoam
-glue

60-90% success rate

IV VASOPRESSIN
-50% rebleeding rate
-ineffective for gastroduodenal artery bleeds

SURGERY

Failure to identify or control bleeding endoscopically

Angiography unavailable

>6U PRBC Tx

Suture-ligation of bleeder vagotomy+pyloroplasty

Bleeding duodenal ulcer

Vagotomy + antrectomy
Ulcer excision

Bleeding gastric ulcer

Further Reading

Barkun AN, Almadi M, Kuipers EJ, et al. Management of nonvariceal upper gastrointestinal bleeding: guideline recommendations from the international consensus group. Ann Intern Med. 2019;171:805.

Communication from the ASGE Standards of Practice Committee. The role of endoscopy in the management of acute non-variceal upper GI bleeding. Gastrointest Endosc. 2012;75:1132–8.

Dultz LA, Lipsett PA. Upper GI bleeding. In: McIntyre Jr RC, Schulick RD, editors. Surgical decision making. 6th ed. Philadelphia: Elsevier; 2020. p. 126–36.

- Lower gastrointestinal bleeding (LGIB) is a common urgent/emergent clinical entity. In the USA approximately 1.7 million cases are reported per year.
- Traditionally, it is defined as bleeding distal to the ligament of Treitz.
- Compared with upper GI bleeding, there are many more etiologies of LGIB. The diagnosis may frequently be elusive due to the intermittent nature of the bleeding. Significant amounts of blood present in the GI tract may hinder endoscopic localization and treatment.
- Benign anorectal causes comprise 5–20% of LGIB and should always be ruled out upon evaluation. Hemorrhoidal disease is a common culprit. Bleeding is rarely massive; chronic iron deficiency anemia is frequently present.
- Infectious colitis is characterized by self-limiting bloody diarrhea. Frequent causative organisms include *Campylobacter, Salmonella, Escherichia coli.*
- Rectal varices are a sequela of cirrhosis and portosystemic shunt. Bleeding varices (as well as hemorrhoidal bleeding) are exacerbated by the associated coagulopathy and may be massive.
- Diverticulosis is the most common cause of massive LGIB (50–90%). Predisposing factors include use/abuse of NSAIDS, hypertension, and antiplatelet/anticoagulant drugs. Bleeding will stop spontaneously in 80% of cases and will recur in 40%.
- Angioectasia (also known as arteriovenous malformation/angiodysplasia) is a cause of LGIB in 3–15% of cases. It may be associated with von Willebrand's disease, chronic renal failure, and aortic stenosis. The cecum and right colon are most commonly affected. Advanced age, multiple lesions, and the use of antiplatelet/anticoagulant drugs are risk factors for LGIB.
- Post-polypectomy LGIB occurs in <1% of interventions but may account for up to 8% of LGIB.
- Colorectal Kaposi sarcoma may cause LGIB in HIV/AIDS patients.
- LGIB is common in patients with ulcerative colitis and Crohn's colitis.

- Colorectal cancer does result in blood loss. However, massive LGIB is rare. The usual clinical manifestation is blood mixed with stool in left colonic/rectal lesions, occult bleeding in right colonic lesions. Tenesmus may be present.
- Ischemic colitis may manifest as bloody stools associated with abdominal pain. It is the result of sloughing of ischemic mucosa. Massive LGIB is rare.
- In general, LGIB with abdominal pain usually indicates **ischemia, infection, or IBD.**
- In 10–15% of massive LGIB, the source may proximal to the ligament of Treitz and should be ruled out. The differential includes gastroduodenal ulcer, esophageal varices, gastric varices, and aortoduodenal fistula.
- The initial management of LGIB starts with the assessment of the patient's hemodynamic status. Massive LGIB may manifest with orthostatic or profound hypotension, tachycardia, chest pain, and shortness of breath. **Remember your ABC's!**
- Two antecubital, large bore (14–16 gauge) IV cannula provide optimal access for fluid resuscitation and blood/component transfusion. A Foley catheter is placed, and noninvasive hemodynamic monitoring is initiated immediately.
- Upper GI bleeding must be ruled out. This is achieved by NG tube placement and aspirate assessment. Bilious material effectively rules out upper GI bleeding. Return of blood/bloody material reveals an upper GI source and should be followed by upper endoscopy. Return of clear fluid cannot rule out upper GI bleeding.
- A CBC, PT/PTT, blood type, and crossmatch are immediately obtained. Transfusion of O negative blood may be necessary when type-matched blood is unavailable.
- The use of certain medications is key during history-taking: NSAIDS, antiplatelet, and anticoagulant medications.
- The onset, frequency, duration of blood passed per rectum is assessed. It may give a clue in localizing the bleeding source:
  - **Bright red blood**: anorectal, left colon

- **Maroon**: right colon, small bowel, massive upper GI bleed
- **Melena**: Upper GI bleed, moderate small bowel bleeding, moderate right colon bleeding.
- Hypovolemia may be assessed by clinical signs. Tachycardia suggests moderate hypovolemia. Orthostatic hypotension suggests a blood volume loss of <15%. Supine hypotension suggests a blood volume loss of >40%
- On physical exam one should carefully look for abdominal scars, assess for pain/tenderness/distension as well as signs of hepatic disease (hepatomegaly, splenomegaly, palmar erythema, caput medusa).
- A digital rectal exam with proctosigmoidoscopy will rule out anorectal causes of LGIB.
- Initial resuscitation includes a crystalloid fluid bolus (0.5–1 lt) with frequent or continuous blood pressure monitoring to assess response. Transfusion thresholds are a Hb <7 mg/dl for younger patients, 9 mg/dl for older patients.
- INR is checked to assess coagulopathy. Component transfusion is initiated when INR >2.5.
- Various diagnostic modalities for LGIB exist with variable accuracy rates. They are utilized depending on the rate of bleeding and institutional availability.
- Radionuclide imaging consists of tagging a patient's RBC with an isotope, reinjecting them, and serially scanning the patient after 30 min. It may detect bleeding at a rate of 0.04–01 ml/min and has an overall accuracy rate of 24–91%. It depicts a generalized area of bleeding. In addition, extravasated blood may move in the GI tract, lowering the precision of bleeding localization. The scan may be positive after the bleeding stops; this is useful in intermittent GI bleeds.
- CT angiography may detect active bleeding (at a rate of 0.3/1 ml/min) with a great degree of accuracy with regards to localization. It can detect coexisting pathology such as a tumor. Reported diagnostic sensitivity is 85–92%.

Radiation exposure, contrast-induced allergic reaction, and contrast-associated nephropathy are adverse sequelae.
- Angiography detects bleeding at a rate of 0.5–1 ml/min. It is an invasive intervention with therapeutic potential. Indications for angiography include hemodynamic instability, transfusion of >5U PRBC, and a 50% drop in Hb. Diagnostic selective angiography is performed by sequential imaging of the SMA, IMA, and celiac axis. Therapeutic angiography can be performed either by infusion of a vasoconstricting agent (e.g., vasopressin) or selective/superselective embolization with coils, gelfoam, or PVC. Intestinal infarction, renal injury, and vascular injury are adverse sequelae.
- Colonoscopy may detect the bleeding source in 74–100% of cases. Rapid bowel preparation via an NG tube is recommended; in addition, blood in colon may facilitate preparation as it acts as a cathartic. Clips, epinephrine, monopolar/bipolar current, and argon plasma may achieve hemostasis. Perforation is an adverse sequela.
- A negative upper GI/colonic bleed evaluation points to a small bowel source. Diagnostic options include video capsule endoscopy, double-balloon enteroscopy, intraoperative enteroscopy, and a Meckel scan.
- Indications for surgery include massive transfusion requirements and hemodynamic instability despite therapeutic efforts. **Ideally, the source must be localized prior to surgery.**
- Surgical maneuvers include:
  - Full exploration of small bowel along the entire length to rule out lesions/Meckel's diverticulum. Bowel transillumination may detect angioectasia
  - Intraoperative colonoscopy, gastroduodenoscopy, enteroscopy.
  - If no source is found a total abdominal colectomy with ileostomy or ileorectostomy can be performed. The rebleeding rate with this approach is approximately 5%. **Blind segmental colonic resections have a much higher rebleeding rate (30–70%).**

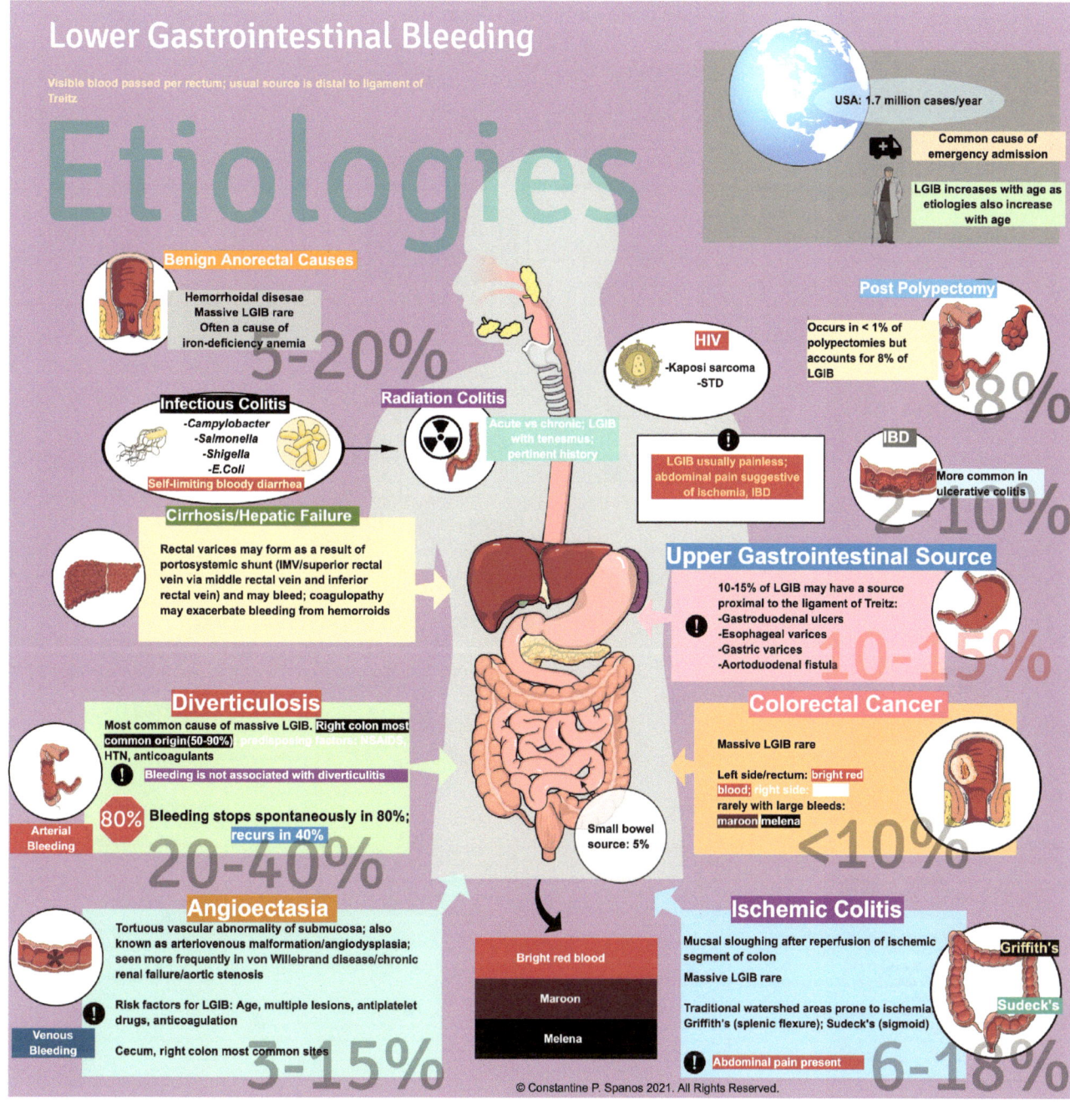

Lower Gastrointestinal Bleeding

Visible blood passed per rectum; usual source is distal to ligament of Treitz

Etiologies

USA: 1.7 million cases/year

Common cause of emergency admission

LGIB increases with age as etiologies also increase with age

Benign Anorectal Causes
Hemorrhoidal disesae
Massive LGIB rare
Often a cause of iron-deficiency anemia

5-20%

Infectious Colitis
-Campylobacter
-Salmonella
-Shigella
-E.Coli
Self-limiting bloody diarrhea

Radiation Colitis
Acute vs chronic; LGIB with tenesmus; pertinent history

HIV
-Kaposi sarcoma
-STD

Post Polypectomy
Occurs in < 1% of polypectomies but accounts for 8% of LGIB

8%

LGIB usually painless; abdominal pain suggestive of ischemia, IBD

IBD
More common in ulcerative colitis

2-10%

Cirrhosis/Hepatic Failure
Rectal varices may form as a result of portosystemic shunt (IMV/superior rectal vein via middle rectal vein and inferior rectal vein) and may bleed; coagulopathy may exacerbate bleeding from hemorrhoids

Upper Gastrointestinal Source
10-15% of LGIB may have a source proximal to the ligament of Treitz:
-Gastroduodenal ulcers
-Esophageal varices
-Gastric varices
-Aortoduodenal fistula

10-15%

Diverticulosis
Most common cause of massive LGIB. Right colon most common origin(50-90%) predisposing factors: NSAIDS, HTN, anticoagulants

Bleeding is not associated with diverticulitis

80% Bleeding stops spontaneously in 80%; recurs in 40%

Arterial Bleeding

20-40%

Colorectal Cancer
Massive LGIB rare

Left side/rectum: bright red blood; right side: rarely with large bleeds: maroon melena

<10%

Small bowel source: 5%

Angioectasia
Tortuous vascular abnormality of submucosa; also known as arteriovenous malformation/angiodysplasia; seen more frequently in von Willebrand disease/chronic renal failure/aortic stenosis

Risk factors for LGIB: Age, multiple lesions, antiplatelet drugs, anticoagulation

Cecum, right colon most common sites

Venous Bleeding

3-15%

Ischemic Colitis
Mucsal sloughing after reperfusion of ischemic segment of colon

Massive LGIB rare

Traditional watershed areas prone to ischemia Griffith's (splenic flexure); Sudeck's (sigmoid)

Abdominal pain present

Griffith's

Sudeck's

6-18%

Bright red blood

Maroon

Melena

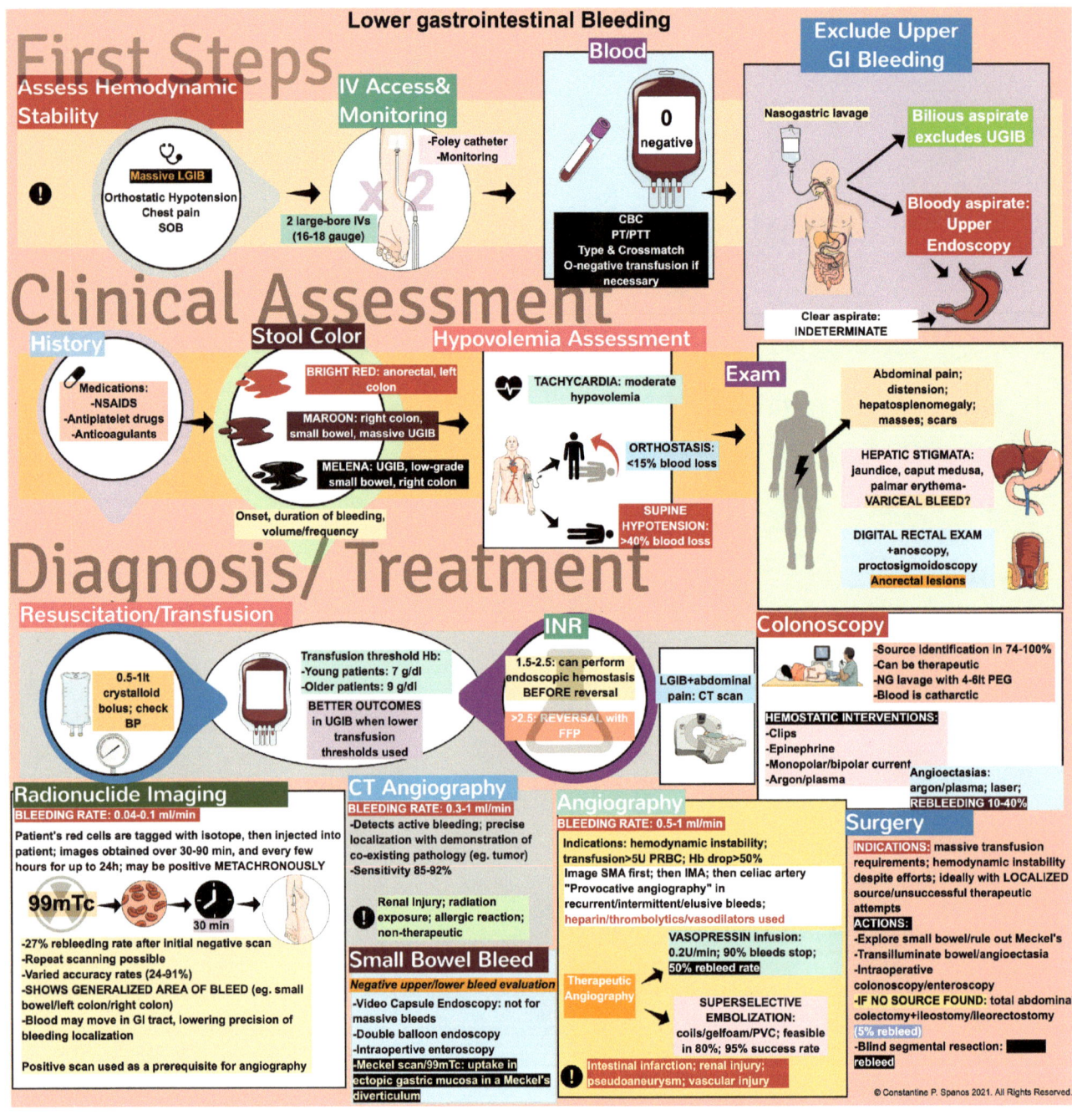

Lower gastrointestinal Bleeding

First Steps

Assess Hemodynamic Stability

Massive LGIB
Orthostatic Hypotension
Chest pain
SOB

IV Access& Monitoring

-Foley catheter
-Monitoring

2 large-bore IVs (16-18 gauge)
x2

Blood

0 negative

CBC
PT/PTT
Type & Crossmatch
O-negative transfusion if necessary

Exclude Upper GI Bleeding

Nasogastric lavage

Bilious aspirate excludes UGIB

Bloody aspirate: Upper Endoscopy

Clear aspirate: INDETERMINATE

Clinical Assessment

History

Medications:
-NSAIDS
-Antiplatelet drugs
-Anticoagulants

Onset, duration of bleeding, volume/frequency

Stool Color

BRIGHT RED: anorectal, left colon

MAROON: right colon, small bowel, massive UGIB

MELENA: UGIB, low-grade small bowel, right colon

Hypovolemia Assessment

TACHYCARDIA: moderate hypovolemia

ORTHOSTASIS: <15% blood loss

SUPINE HYPOTENSION: >40% blood loss

Exam

Abdominal pain; distension; hepatosplenomegaly; masses; scars

HEPATIC STIGMATA: jaundice, caput medusa, palmar erythema- VARICEAL BLEED?

DIGITAL RECTAL EXAM +anoscopy, proctosigmoidoscopy
Anorectal lesions

Diagnosis/ Treatment

Resuscitation/Transfusion

0.5-1lt crystalloid bolus; check BP

Transfusion threshold Hb:
-Young patients: 7 g/dl
-Older patients: 9 g/dl
BETTER OUTCOMES in UGIB when lower transfusion thresholds used

INR

1.5-2.5: can perform endoscopic hemostasis BEFORE reversal

>2.5: REVERSAL with FFP

LGIB+abdominal pain: CT scan

Colonoscopy

-Source identification in 74-100%
-Can be therapeutic
-NG lavage with 4-6lt PEG
-Blood is cathartic

HEMOSTATIC INTERVENTIONS:
-Clips
-Epinephrine
-Monopolar/bipolar current
-Argon/plasma

Angioectasias: argon/plasma; laser; REBLEEDING 10-40%

Radionuclide Imaging

BLEEDING RATE: 0.04-0.1 ml/min

Patient's red cells are tagged with isotope, then injected into patient; images obtained over 30-90 min, and every few hours for up to 24h; may be positive METACHRONOUSLY

99mTc → → 30 min →

-27% rebleeding rate after initial negative scan
-Repeat scanning possible
-Varied accuracy rates (24-91%)
-SHOWS GENERALIZED AREA OF BLEED (eg. small bowel/left colon/right colon)
-Blood may move in GI tract, lowering precision of bleeding localization

Positive scan used as a prerequisite for angiography

CT Angiography

BLEEDING RATE: 0.3-1 ml/min

-Detects active bleeding; precise localization with demonstration of co-existing pathology (eg. tumor)
-Sensitivity 85-92%

Renal Injury; radiation exposure; allergic reaction; non-therapeutic

Small Bowel Bleed

Negative upper/lower bleed evaluation

-Video Capsule Endoscopy: not for massive bleeds
-Double balloon endoscopy
-Intraopertive enteroscopy
-Meckel scan/99mTc: uptake in ectopic gastric mucosa in a Meckel's diverticulum

Angiography

BLEEDING RATE: 0.5-1 ml/min

Indications: hemodynamic instability; transfusion>5U PRBC; Hb drop>50%
Image SMA first; then IMA; then celiac artery
"Provocative angiography" in recurrent/intermittent/elusive bleeds;
heparin/thrombolytics/vasodilators used

Therapeutic Angiography

VASOPRESSIN infusion: 0.2U/min; 90% bleeds stop; 50% rebleed rate

SUPERSELECTIVE EMBOLIZATION: coils/gelfoam/PVC; feasible in 80%; 95% success rate

Intestinal infarction; renal injury; pseudoaneurysm; vascular injury

Surgery

INDICATIONS: massive transfusion requirements; hemodynamic instability despite efforts; ideally with LOCALIZED source/unsuccessful therapeutic attempts

ACTIONS:
-Explore small bowel/rule out Meckel's
-Transilluminate bowel/angioectasia
-Intraoperative colonoscopy/enteroscopy
-IF NO SOURCE FOUND: total abdominal colectomy+ileostomy/ileorectostomy (5% rebleed)
-Blind segmental resection: ▮ rebleed

Further Reading

Kann BR, Vargas HD. Lower gastrointestinal hemorrhage. In: Steele SR, Hull TR, Read TE, Saclarides TJ, Senagore AJ, Whitlow CB, editors. The ASCRS textbook of colon and rectal surgery. 3rd ed. Heidelberg: Springer; 2016. p. 697–716.

Strate LL, Gralnek IM. ACG clinical guideline: management of patients with acute lower gastrointestinal bleeding. Am J Gastroenterol. 2016;111:459.

Wilson AM, Lynch K. The management of lower gastrointestinal bleeding. In: Cameron JL, Cameron AM, editors. Current surgical therapy. 12th ed. Philadelphia: Elsevier; 2017. p. 322–4.

- Esophageal variceal bleeding is a major cause of morbidity and mortality in cirrhotic patients with portal hypertension. Bleeding is often massive.
- The goals of treatment are to restore and maintain hemodynamic stability, restore and maintain oxygenation, control bleeding, and prevent complications.
- Patients with esophageal variceal bleeding are admitted to the ICU. Intubation is often required to protect the airway and prevent aspiration.
- Fluid resuscitation, blood transfusion, and transfusion of plasma/recombinant factor VIIa are frequently required secondary to hepatic clotting factor deficiency.
- Vasoactive drugs are used to mitigate/treat bleeding and restore hemodynamics:
  - Octreotide 25–50 μg/h
  - Vasopressin 0.4 U bolus followed by 0.4–1 U/min ± nitroglycerin.
  - Terlipressin 2 mg IV q 4 h followed by 1 mg IV q 4 h.
  - Hyponatremia, myocardial/organ ischemia are adverse sequelae.
- Antibiotics, namely ciprofloxacin or ceftriaxone, have been associated with reduced rebleeding and infection rates. Mortality also seems to be reduced.
- Endoscopy is performed within 12 h. A small proportion of UGIB in cirrhotic patients is secondary to other causes, such as a Mallory-Weiss tear.
- Endoscopic bleeding control is achieved with banding; several sessions may be required.
- Balloon tamponade can be used for temporary bleeding control. Intubation is often required; there is also a risk of perforation and aspiration. There is a 60% rebleeding rate with this treatment modality.

- Alternatively, endoscopic placement of a self-expanding metal stent has been used for refractory bleeding.
- Transjugular intrahepatic portosystemic shunts (TIPS) have replaced emergency surgery for refractory variceal bleeding. Hemorrhagic control is achieved in 90–100% of cases. It is used selectively in cases of compromised (Child-Pugh B)/decompensated (Child-Pugh C) hepatopathy.
- Surgical shunt procedures include nonselective portacaval shunts, small-diameter H-graft portacaval shunts, mesocaval shunts, and distal splenorenal shunts. **Of note, surgical shunts may complicate future liver transplantation.**
- The modified Sugiura procedure can be performed emergently. It includes esophageal transection, proximal gastric devascularization, and splenectomy. This procedure is rarely performed in the era of TIPS and liver transplantation and has significant morbidity and mortality.
- Liver transplantation is the optimal procedure for decompensated patients (Child-Pugh C) with esophageal varices. It is hindered by donor availability. Compensated (Child-Pugh A)/compromised (Child-Pugh B) patients are usually treated with endoscopic variceal banding until hepatic function deteriorates further.
- Gastric varices are treated with vasoactive drugs, balloon tamponade, cyanoacrylate glue injection, TIPS, banding, and balloon-occluded retrograde transvenous obliteration (BRTO).
- In hepatopathic patients, the Child-Pugh score is utilized to classify patients regarding disease and treatment morbidity/mortality.

Esophageal Variceal Bleeding

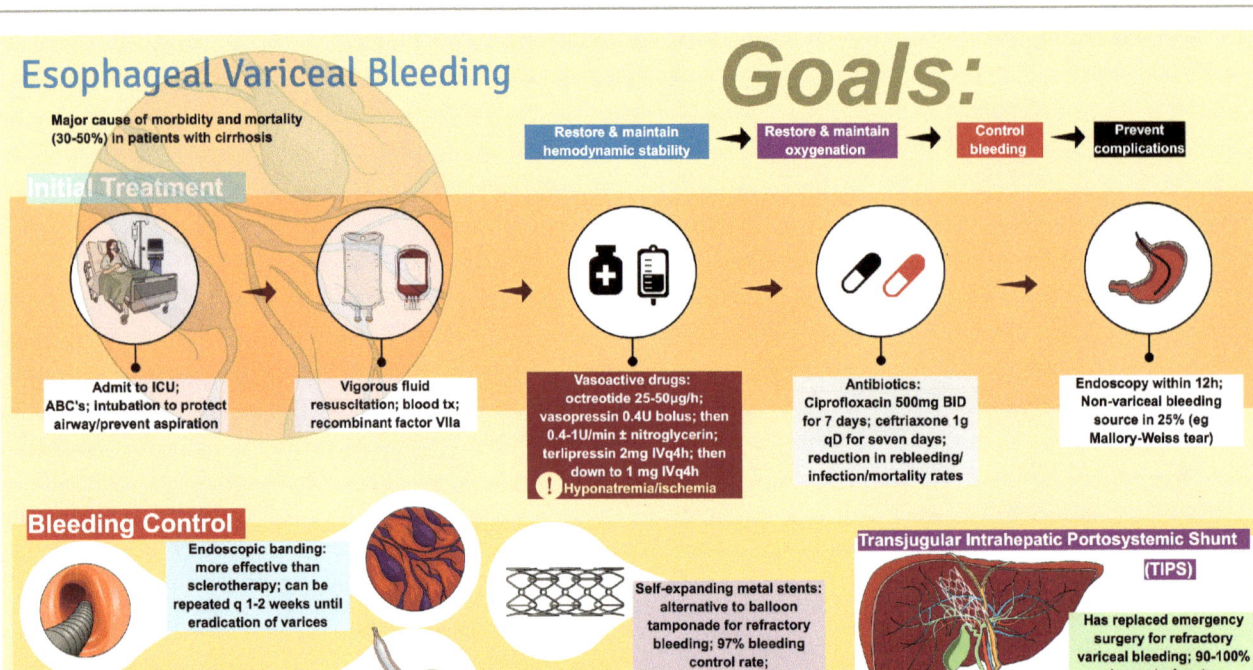

Major cause of morbidity and mortality (30-50%) in patients with cirrhosis

Goals:

Restore & maintain hemodynamic stability → Restore & maintain oxygenation → Control bleeding → Prevent complications

Initial Treatment

Admit to ICU; ABC's; intubation to protect airway/prevent aspiration

Vigorous fluid resuscitation; blood tx; recombinant factor VIIa

Vasoactive drugs: octreotide 25-50µg/h; vasopressin 0.4U bolus; then 0.4-1U/min ± nitroglycerin; terlipressin 2mg IVq4h; then down to 1 mg IVq4h
⚠ Hyponatremia/ischemia

Antibiotics: Ciprofloxacin 500mg BID for 7 days; ceftriaxone 1g qD for seven days; reduction in rebleeding/infection/mortality rates

Endoscopy within 12h; Non-variceal bleeding source in 25% (eg Mallory-Weiss tear)

Bleeding Control

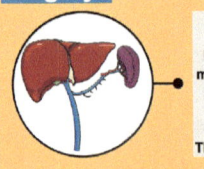

Endoscopic banding: more effective than sclerotherapy; can be repeated q 1-2 weeks until eradication of varices

Balloon tamponade: 80-90% temporary bleeding control rate; 60% re-bleeding rate; PERFORATION /ASPIRATION RISK

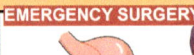

Self-expanding metal stents: alternative to balloon tamponade for refractory bleeding; 97% bleeding control rate; MIGRATION/ULCERATION

Transjugular Intrahepatic Portosystemic Shunt

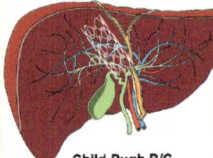

(TIPS)

Has replaced emergency surgery for refractory variceal bleeding; 90-100% hemostasis rate; embolization of feeding esophageal vein possible; 12-20% recurrent bleeding

Child-Pugh B/C SELECTIVELY; Score>13 HIGH MORTALITY

Surgery

Shunt Procedures
Nonselective portacaval shunts; small-diameter H-graft portacaval shunts; mesocaval shunts; selective shunts/distal splenorenal shunts:
AVOID SHUNTS IN LIVER TRANSPLANT CANDIDATES

EMERGENCY SURGERY

Esophageal transection, proximal gastric devascularization, splenectomy; alternatively, central portacaval shunt

Liver Transplantation

Ultimately, liver transplantation is the optimal surgical procedure for Child-Pugh C patients; Child-Pugh A/B treated with endoscopic banding until hepatic function deteriorates further

Gastric Varices

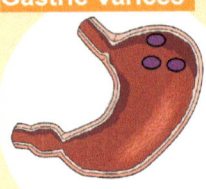

-Vasoactive drugs (octreotide/vasopressin/terlipressin)
-Balloon tamponade
-Cyanoacrylate glue injection
- TIPS
-Banding
-Balloon-occluded retrograde transvenous obliteration (BRTO)

Child-Pugh Score

POINTS	1	2	3
Ascites	absent	slight	moderate
Bilirubin	<2mg/dl	2-3mg/dl	>3mg/dl
Albumin	>3.5 mg/dl	2.8-3.5 mg/dl	<2.8 mg/dl
INR	<1.7	1.7-2.3	>2.3
Encephalopathy	none	Grade 1-2	Grade 3-4

Child-Pugh A: 5-6 (compensated)
Child-Pugh B: 7-9 (compromised)
Child-Pugh C: 10-15 (decompensated)

Further Reading

Kapoor A, Dharel N, Sanyal AJ. Endoscopic diagnosis and therapy in gastroesophageal variceal bleeding. Gastrointest Endosc Clin N Am. 2015;25(3):491–507.

McCarty TR, Njei B. Self-expanding metal stents for acute refractory esophageal variceal bleeding: a systematic review and meta-analysis. Dig Endosc. 2016;28(5):539–47.

Tripathi D, Stanley AJ, Hayes PC, et al. UK guidelines on the management of variceal hemorrhage in cirrhotic patients. Gut. 2015;64:1680.

Van Stiegmann G. Bleeding esophageal varices. In: McIntyre Jr RC, Schulick RD, editors. Surgical decision making. 6th ed. Philadelphia: Elsevier; 2020. p. 138–9.

- Ingestion of caustic substances has the potential for serious morbidity and mortality. The two main categories of ingested substances are alkalis and acids. These cause different types of injury and have a differing distribution of damage.
- Ingestion is most commonly accidental in children, but intentional in adults. Many of these adults have underlying mental health illness.
- **Strong alkalis** (sodium and potassium hydroxide) are found in drain cleaners, household cleaning products, and disc batteries, and are the most common liquid ingested. Alkalis cause **liquefactive** necrosis; there is rapid transmural destruction of esophageal tissue, extending to surrounding mediastinal tissue. In addition, the process may take up to 4 days from ingestion. Ultimately, fibrosis of the esophageal wall may develop, resulting in stricture formation.
- The stomach and duodenum are damaged when a large volume of alkali is ingested.
- **Strong acids** are found in the toilet bowl and swimming pool cleaners (hydrochloric, sulfuric, and phosphoric acid). They cause **coagulation** necrosis. Acids cause pain on ingestion thus preventing large amount from reaching the stomach. Gagging and coughing result in oropharyngeal and upper airway injuries. Esophageal injury is rare.
- It is very important to obtain a careful and detailed history to determine the type and volume of substance ingested.
- Patients may present with chest pain, throat pain, dyspnea, tachypnea, odynophagia emesis, and hematemesis.
- Nasal flaring, drooling stridor, dyspnea, hoarseness, and the presence of subcutaneous emphysema are suggestive of epiglottic injury and laryngeal edema and may constitute an airway emergency.
- Fever, tachycardia, peritonitis, and shock are suggestive of esophageal or gastric perforation.
- Vomiting, chest pain, and subcutaneous emphysema are known as **Mackler's triad** and are suggestive of **esophageal perforation.**

- Airway assessment is paramount (remember the ABCs). Consider nebulized adrenaline, IV steroids to facilitate airway flow. Severe bronchospasm and airway edema may necessitate intubation or emergency tracheostomy.
- Administration of emetics, neutralizing agents is strongly discouraged, as is the passage of a nasogastric (NG) tube.
- Chest and plain abdominal films may depict subcutaneous emphysema, pneumomediastinum, pneumoperitoneum, and pleural effusion.
- CT scan of the chest and abdomen is very useful in determining the depth and extent of esophageal and gastric wall injury. Transmural necrosis with perforation is accurately depicted, prompting emergency surgery. The extent and location of injury to surrounding tissues and anatomical spaces are also depicted.
- Endoscopy is performed to assess injury severity. It should be performed within 24–48 h of ingestion; after this period the risk of iatrogenic perforation is high.
- Endoscopic esophageal injury classification is as follows:
  - 1st degree: superficial mucosal injury; mucosal edema and erythema
  - 2nd degree: submucosal injury; ulceration, exudates, and vesicles
  - 3rd degree: transmural injury; deep ulcers black discoloration, perforation
- Low-grade injuries (1st degree) can be treated with supportive care in an ICU setting. This includes pain control, gastric acid suppression, NPO, parenteral nutrition until pain-free. Psychiatric consultation is advised.
- Esophageal perforation with extensive necrosis is an indication for emergency surgery. A transhiatal esophagectomy (± gastrectomy) with cervical esophagostomy (spit fistula) and feeding jejunostomy is performed. Reestablishing alimentary tract continuity is performed electively later.
- In poor surgical candidates with limited injury/small perforations, an esophageal stent can be placed endoscopically.

- Long-term complications of caustic esophageal injury include strictures, which are frequent. Dilation and bougienage require multiple sessions with varying results. Early stent placement for stricture prevention has been reported, with varying results. Definitive reconstruction (esophagectomy with conduit esophageal replacement may be required).
- Esophageal cancer may develop several decades after injury. Endoscopic surveillance every 2–3 years, starting at 10–20 years after injury, is recommended.

15.1 Esophageal Perforation

- Most esophageal perforations (60–70%) are iatrogenic. They may be the result of endoscopy and endoscopic interventions (biopsy, hemostasis, stent placement, stricture dilation, transesophageal echocardiography). They may occur intraoperatively (surgery for achalasia or gastroesophageal reflux disease, complex head and neck surgery).
- A minority of perforations are spontaneous. Most notable is Boerhaave's syndrome; perforation after a bout of violent and protracted retching associated with alcohol consumption. Other causes of perforation include foreign body penetration, caustic ingestion, cancer, and trauma.
- A careful history will reveal the etiology in the majority of cases (endoscopy, instrumentation, retching, etc.).
- Patients may clinically present with chest pain, shoulder pain, epigastric pain. Nausea and vomiting are invariably present. Fever suggests inflammation of surrounding tissues (cervicitis, mediastinitis, and peritonitis).
- Vomiting, chest pain, and subcutaneous emphysema are known as **Mackler's triad** and are suggestive and characteristic of esophageal perforation.
- Patients are classified as clinically stable or unstable (sepsis, shock).
- Diagnostic investigations include:
  - Labs: CBC, BMP, lactate.
  - Plain films (chest, abdomen): pneumomediastinum, pneumothorax, pleural effusion, subcutaneous emphysema, abnormal cardio-mediastinal contour.
  - Esophagram: depicts esophageal wall irregularity or contrast extravasation. It shows the level of perforation. Gastrografin is preferred; barium may cause severe inflammation when extravasated.
  - CT scan (chest, abdomen) with contrast: very useful in localizing injury, assessing mediastinal and peritoneal injury.
  - Endoscopy: inspection of mucosal integrity, assessment of injury extent, rules out/in malignancy, stent placement.
- Nonoperative therapy may be appropriate for initial therapy in clinically stable patients with small (<1 cm) contained perforations. Nothing-by-mouth (NPO), head of bed elevation >45°, broad-spectrum antibiotics, PPIs, and parenteral nutrition are instituted. Consider antifungal treatment in patients with gastric reflux. Repeat imaging (esophagram/CT with contrast) is performed at 72–96 h.
- Clinical deterioration is an indication of operative therapy.
- Operative therapy is dictated by the level of perforation and the quality of involved tissues.
- Cervical esophageal perforations are approached via an incision anterior and parallel to the sternocleidomastoid muscle (SCM). The middle thyroid vein is ligated and divided and access to the retropharyngeal space is obtained. If the perforation is found, it is primarily repaired. Closed drainage is performed if it is not found. The strap muscles may be used as a buttress of the repair. An esophagram is obtained 5 days after surgery.
- In perforations of the upper 2/3 of the esophagus, a right posterolateral thoracotomy is performed (fifth interspace). The injury is closed in two layers (mucosa/muscularis). An intercostal muscle flap is used to buttress the repair. An esophagram is obtained 5 days after surgery.
- In perforations of the lower 1/3 of the esophagus, a left posterolateral thoracotomy is performed (seventh interspace). The injury is closed in two layers (mucosa/muscularis). An intercostal/diaphragmatic muscle flap is used to buttress the repair. An esophagram is obtained 5 days after surgery.
- In perforations of the abdominal esophagus, an upper midline abdominal incision is performed. If a large hiatal hernia is present a left thoracotomy is preferable. The injury is primarily repaired; the omentum or gastric fundus (Thal-Dor repair) is used to buttress the repair. Fluoroscopy is performed (esophagogastrogram) 5 days after surgery.
- Unstable patients in septic shock may benefit from performing cervical esophagostomy (spit fistula), distal esophageal occlusion, and a feeding jejunostomy. Subsequent definitive repair is performed electively at a later date.
- An esophageal stent may be used for the repair of small (<1 cm) iatrogenic perforations, in Boerhaave's syndrome and anastomotic leaks. Stents may migrate, perforate, lead to fistula or stricture formation.
- Perforation after dilation of esophageal achalasia is approached via a left anterolateral thoracotomy. Esophagogastric myotomy is performed opposite the perforation. The gastric fundus (Dor-Toupet repair) is used to buttress the repair. Fluoroscopy is performed (esophagogastrogram) 5 days after surgery.
- Esophageal perforation after Nissen fundoplication is treated by unwrapping the fundoplication, primary repair of injury, and redo Nissen fundoplication. Fluoroscopy is performed (esophagogastrogram) 5 days after surgery.

Caustic Esophageal Injury

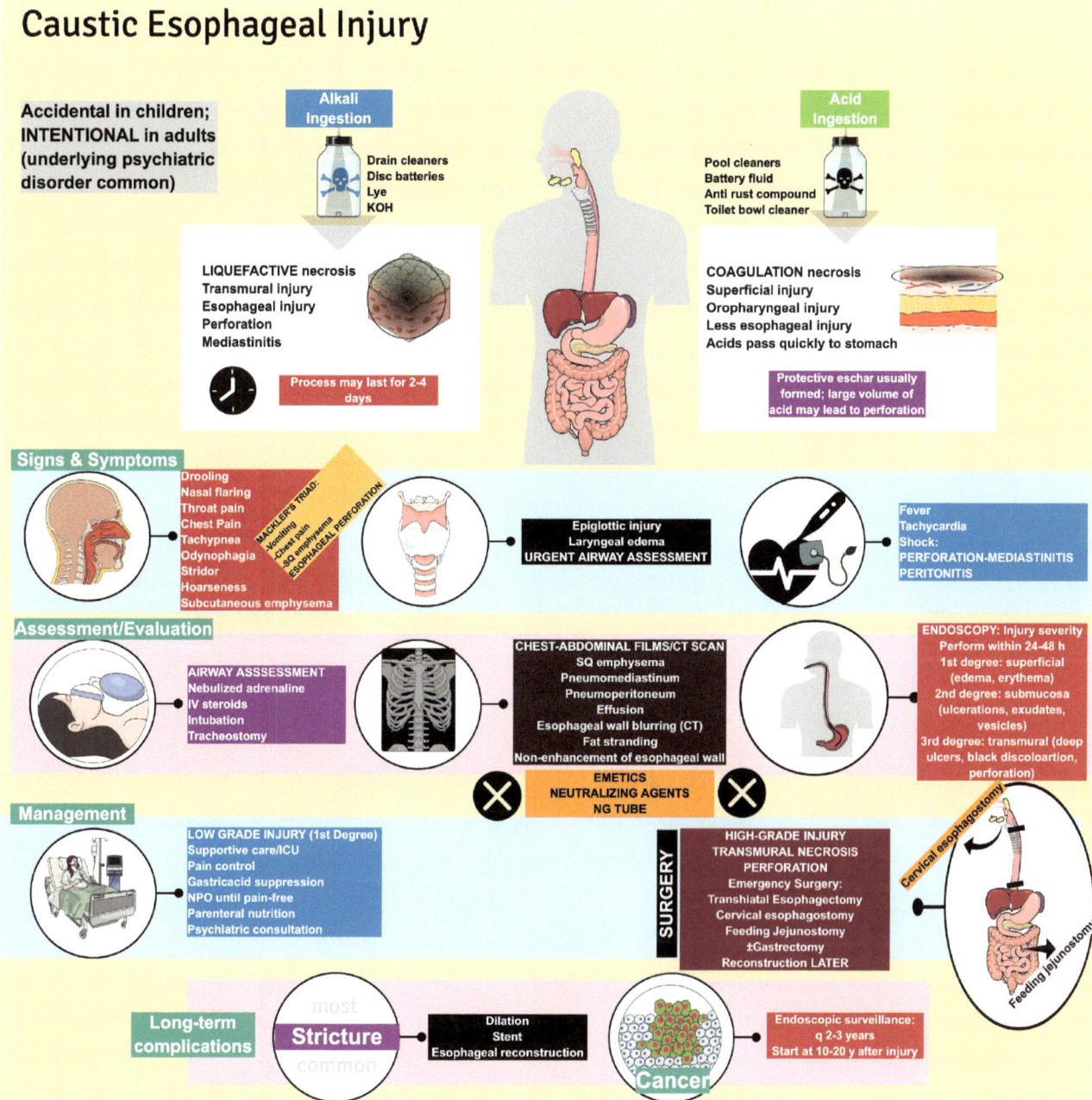

Accidental in children; INTENTIONAL in adults (underlying psychiatric disorder common)

Alkali Ingestion
Drain cleaners
Disc batteries
Lye
KOH

LIQUEFACTIVE necrosis
Transmural injury
Esophageal injury
Perforation
Mediastinitis

Process may last for 2-4 days

Acid Ingestion
Pool cleaners
Battery fluid
Anti rust compound
Toilet bowl cleaner

COAGULATION necrosis
Superficial injury
Oropharyngeal injury
Less esophageal injury
Acids pass quickly to stomach

Protective eschar usually formed; large volume of acid may lead to perforation

Signs & Symptoms
Drooling
Nasal flaring
Throat pain
Chest Pain
Tachypnea
Odynophagia
Stridor
Hoarseness
Subcutaneous emphysema

MACKLER'S TRIAD:
-Vomiting
-Chest pain
-SQ emphysema
ESOPHAGEAL PERFORATION

Epiglottic injury
Laryngeal edema
URGENT AIRWAY ASSESSMENT

Fever
Tachycardia
Shock:
PERFORATION-MEDIASTINITIS
PERITONITIS

Assessment/Evaluation
AIRWAY ASSSESSMENT
Nebulized adrenaline
IV steroids
Intubation
Tracheostomy

CHEST-ABDOMINAL FILMS/CT SCAN
SQ emphysema
Pneumomediastinum
Pneumoperitoneum
Effusion
Esophageal wall blurring (CT)
Fat stranding
Non-enhancement of esophageal wall

ENDOSCOPY: Injury severity
Perform within 24-48 h
1st degree: superficial (edema, erythema)
2nd degree: submucosa (ulcerations, exudates, vesicles)
3rd degree: transmural (deep ulcers, black discoloartion, perforation)

⊗ EMETICS
NEUTRALIZING AGENTS
NG TUBE ⊗

Management
LOW GRADE INJURY (1st Degree)
Supportive care/ICU
Pain control
Gastricacid suppression
NPO until pain-free
Parenteral nutrition
Psychiatric consultation

SURGERY

HIGH-GRADE INJURY
TRANSMURAL NECROSIS
PERFORATION
Emergency Surgery:
Transhiatal Esophagectomy
Cervical esophagostomy
Feeding Jejunostomy
±Gastrectomy
Reconstruction LATER

Cervical esophagostomy

Feeding Jejunostomy

Long-term complications

most
Stricture
common

Dilation
Stent
Esophageal reconstruction

Endoscopic surveillance:
q 2-3 years
Start at 10-20 y after injury

Cancer

Esophageal Perforation

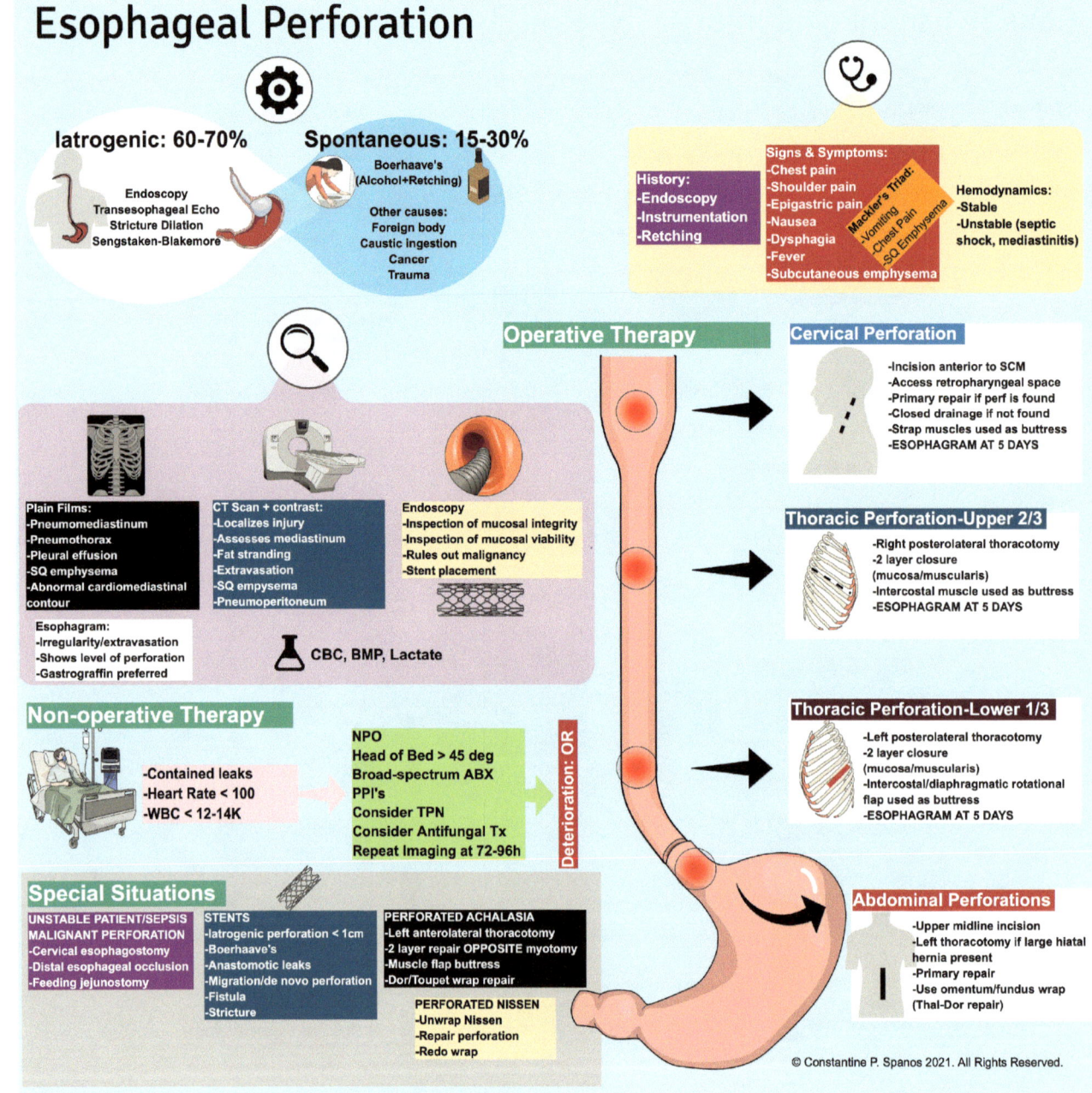

Iatrogenic: 60-70%

Endoscopy
Transesophageal Echo
Stricture Dilation
Sengstaken-Blakemore

Spontaneous: 15-30%

Boerhaave's
(Alcohol+Retching)

Other causes:
Foreign body
Caustic ingestion
Cancer
Trauma

History:
-Endoscopy
-Instrumentation
-Retching

Signs & Symptoms:
-Chest pain
-Shoulder pain
-Epigastric pain
-Nausea
-Dysphagia
-Fever
-Subcutaneous emphysema

Mackler's Triad:
-Vomiting
-Chest Pain
-SQ Emphysema

Hemodynamics:
-Stable
-Unstable (septic shock, mediastinitis)

Plain Films:
-Pneumomediastinum
-Pneumothorax
-Pleural effusion
-SQ emphysema
-Abnormal cardiomediastinal contour

Esophagram:
-Irregularity/extravasation
-Shows level of perforation
-Gastrograffin preferred

CT Scan + contrast:
-Localizes injury
-Assesses mediastinum
-Fat stranding
-Extravasation
-SQ empyema
-Pneumoperitoneum

Endoscopy
-Inspection of mucosal integrity
-Inspection of mucosal viability
-Rules out malignancy
-Stent placement

CBC, BMP, Lactate

Operative Therapy

Cervical Perforation
-Incision anterior to SCM
-Access retropharyngeal space
-Primary repair if perf is found
-Closed drainage if not found
-Strap muscles used as buttress
-ESOPHAGRAM AT 5 DAYS

Thoracic Perforation-Upper 2/3
-Right posterolateral thoracotomy
-2 layer closure (mucosa/muscularis)
-Intercostal muscle used as buttress
-ESOPHAGRAM AT 5 DAYS

Thoracic Perforation-Lower 1/3
-Left posterolateral thoracotomy
-2 layer closure (mucosa/muscularis)
-Intercostal/diaphragmatic rotational flap used as buttress
-ESOPHAGRAM AT 5 DAYS

Non-operative Therapy

-Contained leaks
-Heart Rate < 100
-WBC < 12-14K

NPO
Head of Bed > 45 deg
Broad-spectrum ABX
PPI's
Consider TPN
Consider Antifungal Tx
Repeat Imaging at 72-96h

Deterioration: OR

Abdominal Perforations
-Upper midline incision
-Left thoracotomy if large hiatal hernia present
-Primary repair
-Use omentum/fundus wrap (Thal-Dor repair)

Special Situations

UNSTABLE PATIENT/SEPSIS MALIGNANT PERFORATION
-Cervical esophagostomy
-Distal esophageal occlusion
-Feeding jejunostomy

STENTS
-Iatrogenic perforation < 1cm
-Boerhaave's
-Anastomotic leaks
-Migration/de novo perforation
-Fistula
-Stricture

PERFORATED ACHALASIA
-Left anterolateral thoracotomy
-2 layer repair OPPOSITE myotomy
-Muscle flap buttress
-Dor/Toupet wrap repair

PERFORATED NISSEN
-Unwrap Nissen
-Repair perforation
-Redo wrap

Further Reading

Cheng HT, Cheng CL, Lin CH, et al. Caustic ingestion in adults: the role of endoscopic classification in predicting outcome. BMC Gastroenterol. 2008;8:31.

Maxwell R, Reynolds JK. The management of esophageal perforation. In: Cameron JL, Cameron AM, editors. Current surgical therapy. 12th ed. Philadelphia: Elsevier; 2017. p. 73–8.

Ogburn E, Zwischenberger BA, Miller JD, Zwischenberger JB. Caustic ingestion. In: McIntyre Jr RC, Schulick RD, editors. Surgical decision making. 6th ed. Philadelphia: Elsevier; 2020. p. 110.

- Neutropenic enterocolitis (NE) is a necrotizing enterocolitis secondary to cytotoxic therapy for hematological malignancies. It can affect any portion of the gastrointestinal tract; the colon is most commonly affected. The entity was originally described in children undergoing induction therapy for acute leukemia.
- Cytotoxic drugs may cause bowel mucosal injury and profound neutropenia. As a result, enteric flora invades the systemic circulation, leading to bacteremia and fungemia. The clinical manifestations of neutropenic enterocolitis are a combination of local bowel injury and systemic sepsis.
- Risk factors, or the most common malignancies associated with NE, include acute myelogenic leukemia, lymphoma, multiple myeloma, myelodysplastic syndrome, aplastic anemia as well as immunosuppression, and AIDS.
- Drugs commonly associated with NE include taxanes, cytarabine, 5-FU, capecitabine, cyclophosphamide, ifosfamide, cisplatin, and carboplatin.
- Bowel pathology is characterized by bowel wall thickening infiltrated by bacteria/fungi, mucosal edema, isolated or confluent mucosal ulcers, hemorrhage, or necrosis.
- Abdominal pain with fever and right lower quadrant tenderness (called typhlitis) are common. Patients frequently have watery/bloody diarrhea. Symptoms occur at the third week of cytotoxic therapy. Neutropenia, with an absolute neutrophil count <500/μL, is pathognomonic.
- The differential diagnosis includes acute appendicitis, graft-versus-host disease, ischemic colitis, CMV colitis, and Ogilvie's syndrome.

- CT scan depicts pathological findings such as bowel wall thickening with mucosal enhancement, pneumatosis intestinalis, mesenteric fat stranding, and bowel dilatation.
- Stool cultures may be obtained to rule out infectious colitis; toxin assays/PCR to rule out *Clostridioides Difficile* colitis.
- The initial management of NE includes bowel rest, IV fluids, and nutritional support. In severe cases, NG tube is placed to prevent air accumulation in GI tract.
- Broad spectrum IV antibiotic therapy is initiated, and may include:
  - Piperacillin/tazobactam
  - Cefepime + metronidazole
  - Imipenem/cilastatin
  - Meropenem
  - Enterococcal coverage in severely ill patients
  - Antifungal therapy in patients with persistent fever despite antibiotic therapy
- Transition to oral antibiotics is feasible when patients are nonfebrile for 2 consecutive days and their neutrophil count is >500/μL.
- Bloody diarrhea should prompt evaluation of PT/PTT for coagulopathy and should be corrected accordingly.
- Indications for surgery include perforation/peritonitis, GI bleeding despite support and coagulopathy treatment, and further clinical deterioration. Subtotal colectomy with end-ileostomy may be required. Operation is fraught with high morbidity and mortality.

© The Author(s), under exclusive license to Springer Nature Switzerland AG 2021
C. P. Spanos, *Acute Surgical Topics*, https://doi.org/10.1007/978-3-030-68700-7_16

Neutropenic Enterocolitis

Necrotizing enterocolitis which occurs in neutropenic patients, usually as a result of cytotoxic therapy for hematological malignancies. Originally reported in children undergoing inducton chemotherapy for acute leukemia

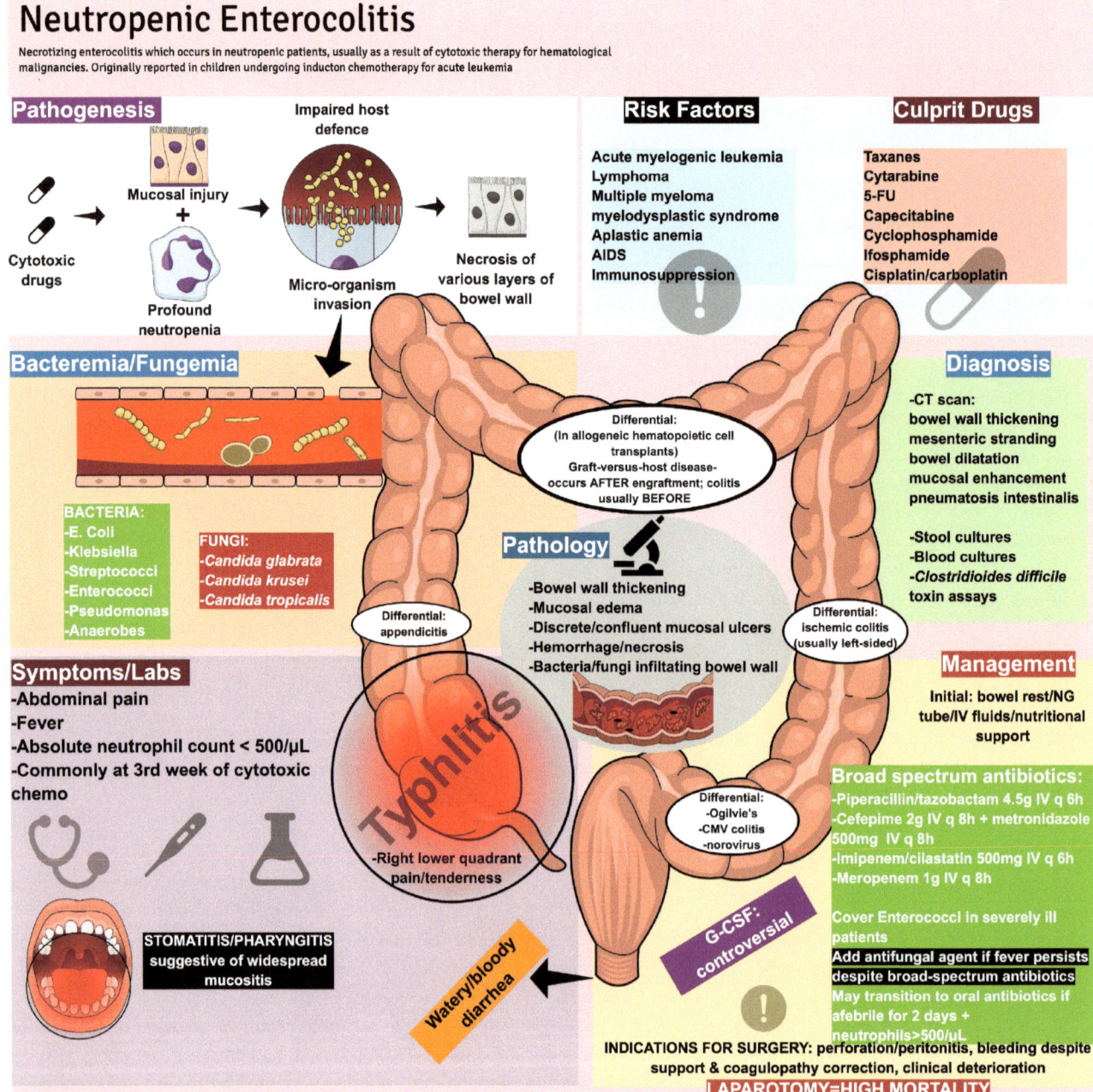

Pathogenesis

Cytotoxic drugs → Mucosal injury + Profound neutropenia → Impaired host defence → Micro-organism invasion → Necrosis of various layers of bowel wall

Risk Factors

Acute myelogenic leukemia
Lymphoma
Multiple myeloma
myelodysplastic syndrome
Aplastic anemia
AIDS
Immunosuppression

Culprit Drugs

Taxanes
Cytarabine
5-FU
Capecitabine
Cyclophosphamide
Ifosphamide
Cisplatin/carboplatin

Bacteremia/Fungemia

BACTERIA:
-E. Coli
-Klebsiella
-Streptococci
-Enterococci
-Pseudomonas
-Anaerobes

FUNGI:
-*Candida glabrata*
-*Candida krusei*
-*Candida tropicalis*

Differential:
(In allogeneic hematopoietic cell transplants)
Graft-versus-host disease-occurs AFTER engraftment; colitis usually BEFORE

Diagnosis

-CT scan:
bowel wall thickening
mesenteric stranding
bowel dilatation
mucosal enhancement
pneumatosis intestinalis

-Stool cultures
-Blood cultures
-*Clostridioides difficile* toxin assays

Pathology

-Bowel wall thickening
-Mucosal edema
-Discrete/confluent mucosal ulcers
-Hemorrhage/necrosis
-Bacteria/fungi infiltating bowel wall

Differential: appendicitis

Differential: ischemic colitis (usually left-sided)

Typhlitis

-Right lower quadrant pain/tenderness

Symptoms/Labs

-Abdominal pain
-Fever
-Absolute neutrophil count < 500/μL
-Commonly at 3rd week of cytotoxic chemo

STOMATITIS/PHARYNGITIS suggestive of widespread mucositis

Differential:
-Ogilvie's
-CMV colitis
-norovirus

Watery/bloody diarrhea

Management

Initial: bowel rest/NG tube/IV fluids/nutritional support

Broad spectrum antibiotics:
-Piperacillin/tazobactam 4.5g IV q 6h
-Cefepime 2g IV q 8h + metronidazole 500mg IV q 8h
-Imipenem/cilastatin 500mg IV q 6h
-Meropenem 1g IV q 8h

Cover Enterococci in severely ill patients
Add antifungal agent if fever persists despite broad-spectrum antibiotics
May transition to oral antibiotics if afebrile for 2 days + neutrophils>500/uL

G-CSF: controversial

INDICATIONS FOR SURGERY: perforation/peritonitis, bleeding despite support & coagulopathy correction, clinical deterioration
LAPAROTOMY=HIGH MORTALITY

Further Reading

Cunningham SC, Fakhry K, Bass BL, et al. Neutropenic enterocolitis in adults: case series and a review of the literature. Dig Dis Sci. 2005;50:215.

Quigley MM, Bethel K, Nowacki M, et al. Neutropenic enterocolitis: a rare presenting complication of acute leukemia. Am J Hematol. 2001;66:213.

Wagner ML, Rosenberg HS, Fernbach DJ, et al. Typhlitis: a complication of leukemia in childhood. Am J Roentgenol Radium Ther Nucl Med. 1970;109:341.

- Acute mesenteric ischemia may prove to be an elusive diagnosis. This is made more complex given the extensive differential diagnosis of acute abdominal pain. Timely diagnosis of mesenteric ischemia requires a high index of suspicion. If left untreated, mortality is 100%.
- Risk factors include advanced age, atherosclerosis, cardiac dysrhythmias, female sex, and hypercoagulability.
- Etiologies include arterial embolism, arterial thrombosis, venous occlusion, and nonocclusive disorders.
- **Mesenteric arterial embolism** is the most frequent cause of acute mesenteric ischemia (40–50%). The origin of emboli are the left cardiac chambers in most cases (clots formed by atrial fibrillation or recent myocardial infarction).
- **Mesenteric arterial thrombosis** is a sequela of atheromatous mesenteric disease. It occurs in 20–35% of cases.
- **Mesenteric venous occlusion/thrombosis** results from hypercoagulable states, inflammatory bowel disease, and trauma. It occurs in 5–15% of cases.
- **Nonocclusive mesenteric ischemia** occurs in low-flow states (after myocardial infarction and heart failure, hemodialysis), mesenteric vasospasm (secondary to vasopressors and cocaine abuse, extreme physical exertion).
- Hypercoagulable states may be inherited, secondary to recent surgery, cancer, or certain drugs (contraceptives, anabolic steroids). Heparin-induced thrombocytopenia may also cause hypercoagulability.
- The classic clinical presentation of acute mesenteric ischemia includes pain out of proportion to clinical findings, namely, severe abdominal pain with few if any peritoneal signs.
- Plain abdominal films may demonstrate pneumoperitoneum, portal venous gas, bowel wall thickening, and pneumatosis intestinalis.
- Ultrasound may demonstrate mesenteric thrombosis and diminished blood flow.
- CT-angiography is the imaging modality with the highest sensitivity/specificity rate (>90%). Mesenteric vascular lesions, bowel wall ischemia, and perforation can be detected.
- Once the diagnosis of mesenteric ischemia is established, anticoagulation is initiated, and broad-spectrum antibiotics are given. Bowel viability should be assessed, and revascularization planned.
- If bowel infarction is unlikely, endovascular/nonoperative treatment may be attempted when extensive expertise exists. This includes suction embolectomy + anticoagulation (for arterial embolism), catheter-directed thrombolysis + stent placement (for arterial thrombosis), anticoagulation ± thrombectomy/thrombolysis (for venous occlusion) and fluid resuscitation, vasodilatory drugs + anticoagulation for nonocclusive disease.
- The threshold for performing exploratory laparotomy should be very low. **Most cases of mesenteric ischemia will require operative exploration.**
- When preparing for laparotomy, harvest of the greater saphenous vein should be anticipated for use as a bypass conduit.
- Operative assessment of bowel viability is key; IV fluorescein, Doppler interrogation of mesenteric vessels, and indocyanine green (ICG) are useful adjuncts in assessing bowel perfusion.
- Mesenteric embolism is characterized by patchy or continuous small bowel ischemia with sparing of the proximal jejunum. A mid-SMA transverse arteriotomy, embolectomy, and patch repair are performed. Infarcted bowel is resected; questionable bowel may be reevaluated with a second-look laparotomy at 24–48 h. Anastomoses may or may not be constructed at initial operation.
- SMA thrombosis is characterized by continuous ischemia/necrosis from proximal jejunum to mid transverse colon. The duodenum is spared. Revascularization is achieved with aorto-mesenteric bypass. The supraceliac or infrarenal aorta, as well as the iliac arteries, may be selected for proximal anastomosis. Infarcted bowel is resected; questionable bowel may be reevaluated with a

C. P. Spanos, *Acute Surgical Topics*, https://doi.org/10.1007/978-3-030-68700-7_17

second-look laparotomy at 24–48 h. Anastomoses may or may not be constructed at initial operation.

- Postoperatively, patients are monitored in an ICU setting. Reperfusion syndrome is not uncommon and increases morbidity/mortality. Abdominal compartment syndrome is also not uncommon. Broad-spectrum antibiotics and anticoagulation are continued.
- Second-look laparotomy (24–48 h after initial exploration) provides reassessment of bowel viability. Further resection may be needed. Bowel anastomoses may be performed if appropriate.
- Usually, lifelong anticoagulation is given in cases of embolism/thrombosis; lifelong antiplatelet treatment is given after bypass procedures and stent placement.
- Short gut syndrome is a serious sequela of mesenteric ischemia and extensive bowel infarction, necessitating lifelong TPN.

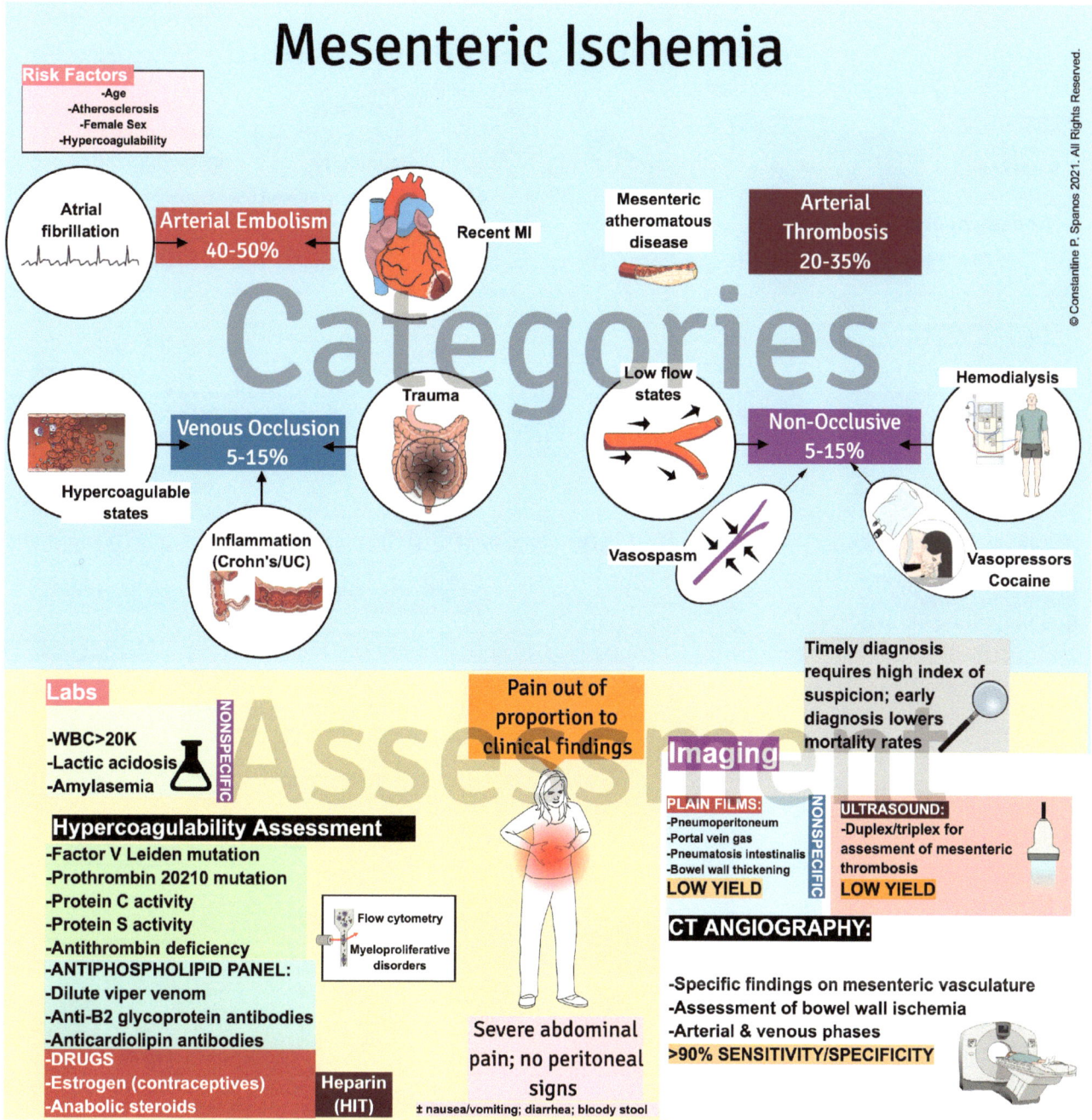

Mesenteric Ischemia

Risk Factors
-Age
-Atherosclerosis
-Female Sex
-Hypercoagulability

Atrial fibrillation

Arterial Embolism 40-50%

Recent MI

Mesenteric atheromatous disease

Arterial Thrombosis 20-35%

Categories

Trauma

Low flow states

Non-Occlusive 5-15%

Hemodialysis

Hypercoagulable states

Venous Occlusion 5-15%

Inflammation (Crohn's/UC)

Vasospasm

Vasopressors Cocaine

Assessment

Labs NONSPECIFIC

-WBC>20K
-Lactic acidosis
-Amylasemia

Hypercoagulability Assessment

-Factor V Leiden mutation
-Prothrombin 20210 mutation
-Protein C activity
-Protein S activity
-Antithrombin deficiency
-ANTIPHOSPHOLIPID PANEL:
-Dilute viper venom
-Anti-B2 glycoprotein antibodies
-Anticardiolipin antibodies
-DRUGS
-Estrogen (contraceptives)
-Anabolic steroids

Flow cytometry
Myeloproliferative disorders

Heparin (HIT)

Pain out of proportion to clinical findings

Severe abdominal pain; no peritoneal signs
± nausea/vomiting; diarrhea; bloody stool

Timely diagnosis requires high index of suspicion; early diagnosis lowers mortality rates

Imaging

PLAIN FILMS: NONSPECIFIC
-Pneumoperitoneum
-Portal vein gas
-Pneumatosis intestinalis
-Bowel wall thickening
LOW YIELD

ULTRASOUND:
-Duplex/triplex for assesment of mesenteric thrombosis
LOW YIELD

CT ANGIOGRAPHY:

-Specific findings on mesenteric vasculature
-Assessment of bowel wall ischemia
-Arterial & venous phases
>90% SENSITIVITY/SPECIFICITY

Mesenteric Ischemia: Treatment

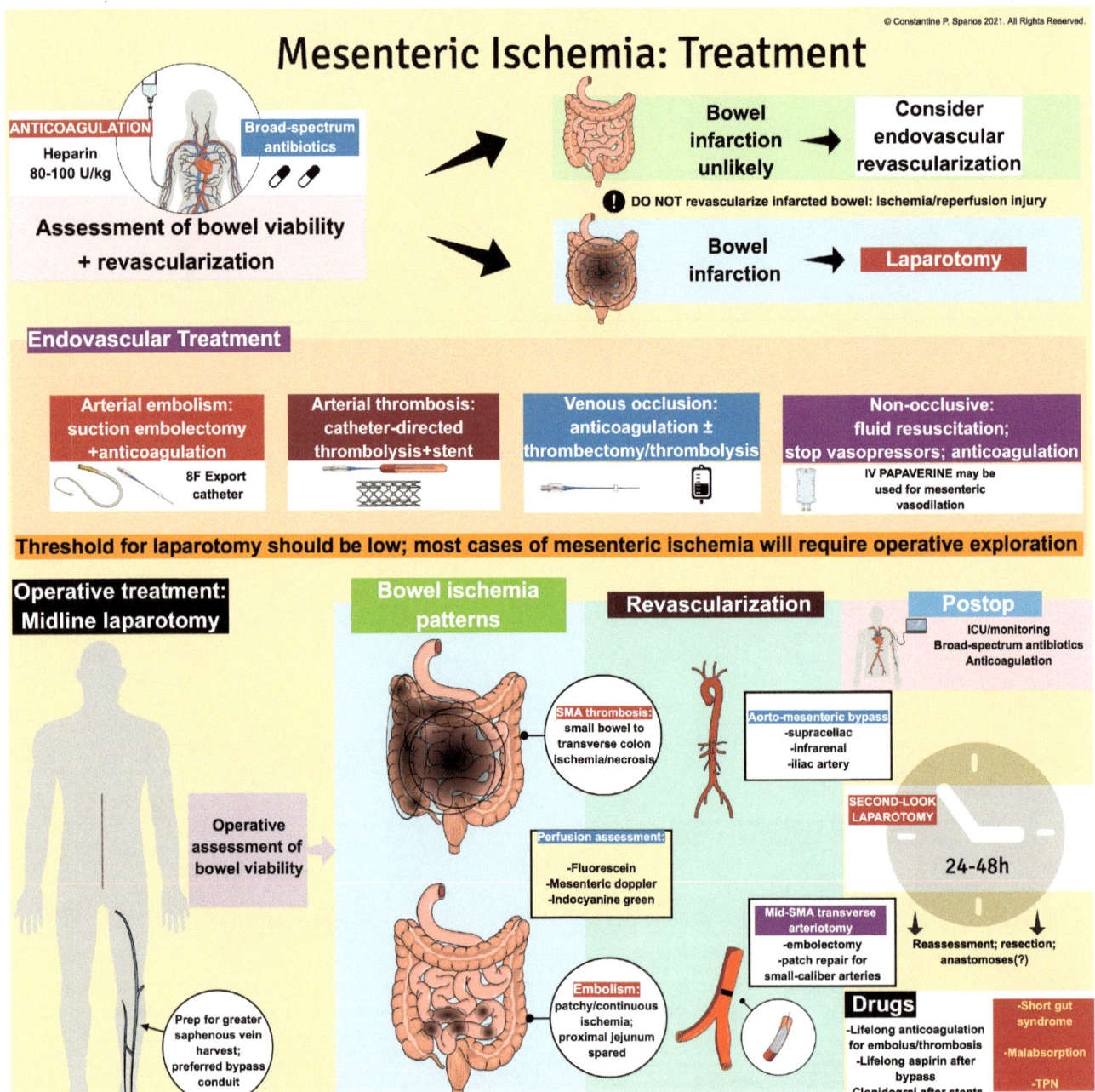

ANTICOAGULATION
Heparin
80-100 U/kg

Broad-spectrum antibiotics

Assessment of bowel viability + revascularization

Bowel infarction unlikely → **Consider endovascular revascularization**

❗ DO NOT revascularize infarcted bowel: Ischemia/reperfusion injury

Bowel infarction → **Laparotomy**

Endovascular Treatment

Arterial embolism: suction embolectomy +anticoagulation
8F Export catheter

Arterial thrombosis: catheter-directed thrombolysis+stent

Venous occlusion: anticoagulation ± thrombectomy/thrombolysis

Non-occlusive: fluid resuscitation; stop vasopressors; anticoagulation
IV PAPAVERINE may be used for mesenteric vasodilation

Threshold for laparotomy should be low; most cases of mesenteric ischemia will require operative exploration

Operative treatment: Midline laparotomy

Bowel ischemia patterns

Revascularization

Postop
ICU/monitoring
Broad-spectrum antibiotics
Anticoagulation

Operative assessment of bowel viability

SMA thrombosis: small bowel to transverse colon ischemia/necrosis

Aorto-mesenteric bypass
-supraceliac
-infrarenal
-iliac artery

Perfusion assessment:
-Fluorescein
-Mesenteric doppler
-Indocyanine green

SECOND-LOOK LAPAROTOMY

24-48h

Mid-SMA transverse arteriotomy
-embolectomy
-patch repair for small-caliber arteries

Reassessment; resection; anastomoses(?)

Prep for greater saphenous vein harvest; preferred bypass conduit

Embolism: patchy/continuous ischemia; proximal jejunum spared

Drugs
-Lifelong anticoagulation for embolus/thrombosis
-Lifelong aspirin after bypass
-Clopidogrel after stents

-Short gut syndrome
-Malabsorption
-TPN

Infarcted bowel resected; questionable bowel re-evaluated with second-look laparotomy

Further Reading

Black JH III, Holscher CM. Acute mesenteric vascular occlusion. In: McIntyre Jr RC, Schulick RD, editors. Surgical decision making. 6th ed. Philadelphia: Elsevier; 2020. p. 174–6.

Eslami MH. Acute mesenteric ischemia. In: Cameron JL, Cameron AM, editors. Current surgical therapy. 12th ed. Philadelphia: Elsevier; 2017. p. 1071–9.

- Abdominal aortic aneurysms (AAA) are relatively common. Rupture of AAA can be one of the most dramatic acute surgical problems. It is associated with up to 80% mortality. A majority of patients die before reaching hospital. Timely diagnosis and expeditious operative treatment have the potential to reduce mortality rates; currently, patients able to reach the operating room have a 30% mortality rate (previously 50%).
- The risk of AAA rupture is proportional to the aneurysm's diameter:
  - Less than 0.5% per year for AAA <4 cm in diameter
  - Approximately 1% per year for AAA 4–5.5 cm in diameter
  - Approximately >3% per year for AAA >5.5 cm in diameter
- Free rupture into the peritoneal cavity often leads to death. Contained rupture leads to temporary tamponade and "buys time" for possible evaluation and treatment if hemodynamic stability is maintained.
- The classic clinical presentation triad of ruptured AAA is hypotension, abdominal pain, and a palpable pulsatile mass. These findings are not always present.
- Hypotension/cardiovascular collapse may be the only clinical manifestation.
- Abdominal pain is often severe, unrelenting, and patients have a sense of impending doom. It often radiates to the back and may extend to the flanks. Abdominal/back pain in a patient with a known AAA is highly suspicious for AAA rupture and warrants prompt investigation.
- Loss of lower extremity peripheral pulses is a frequent finding.
- A palpable pulsatile mass is found in thinner patients with a large AAA.
- In a patient with suspected ruptured AAA, emergency abdominal ultrasound confirms the diagnosis.
- Initial management consists of optimal IV access, type, and crossmatch, with provision for massive blood transfusion as well as platelets and FFP. Permissive hypotension (SBP 80–100 mmg) is preferable.

- **Hemodynamically unstable patients must go to the operating room without imaging.**
- Hemodynamically stable patients can be evaluated with imaging under optimal monitoring since rapid deterioration can occur at any time.
- CT angiography may depict findings of rupture/impending rupture, such as periaortic stranding and retroperitoneal hematoma. It may also provide useful information for operative planning as well as identification of other causes of abdominal pain.
- Once in the OR, the goal is effective hemorrhage control with proximal aortic control.
- Operative open or endovascular approach is selected according to surgeon experience and available institutional resources.
- With an open approach, proximal aortic control is achieved by supraceliac clamping of the aorta via midline laparotomy, or supradiaphragmatic aortic clamping via 5th interspace left thoracotomy. After initial proximal control, the clamp must be placed more distally to prevent visceral ischemia.
- With an endovascular approach, proximal aortic control is achieved with balloon occlusion via bilateral groin access under ultrasound guidance. Angiography is used for endograft deployment. General anesthesia is not required for endovascular repair. In addition, tamponade can be sustained, hemodynamic stability maintained, and fluid shifts, temperature changes, and postoperative ileus avoided. Studies show that there is a decrease in complication rates as well as better survival compared with the open approach.
- Even technically successful repair of ruptured AAA is fraught with high morbidity and mortality. Early mortality is due to bleeding, hemorrhagic shock, and coagulopathy. Late mortality is secondary to sepsis.
- After repair, myocardial infarction occurs in 25–39%, renal failure in 11.5–20%, and respiratory failure in 30–40%.

C. P. Spanos, *Acute Surgical Topics*, https://doi.org/10.1007/978-3-030-68700-7_18

- Lower extremity ischemia is secondary to embolization or occlusion of reconstruction/vascular anastomoses. Endograft kinking/compression may have a similar effect.
- Colon ischemia results from mesenteric vascular occlusion/division. It may manifest as ischemic colitis or colonic infarction. Mild cases are treated with perfusion optimization and antibiotics. Severe cases ± perforation mandate laparotomy, resection, and end-colostomy (Hartmann's), and are associated with high mortality.
- Abdominal compartment syndrome is a serious sequela of ruptured AAA and repair. Etiologies include retroperitoneal hematoma, ongoing bleeding, and bowel edema. It may lead to respiratory distress, renal failure, and shock. In severe cases, decompressive laparotomy is required.

Ruptured Abdominal Aortic Aneurysm

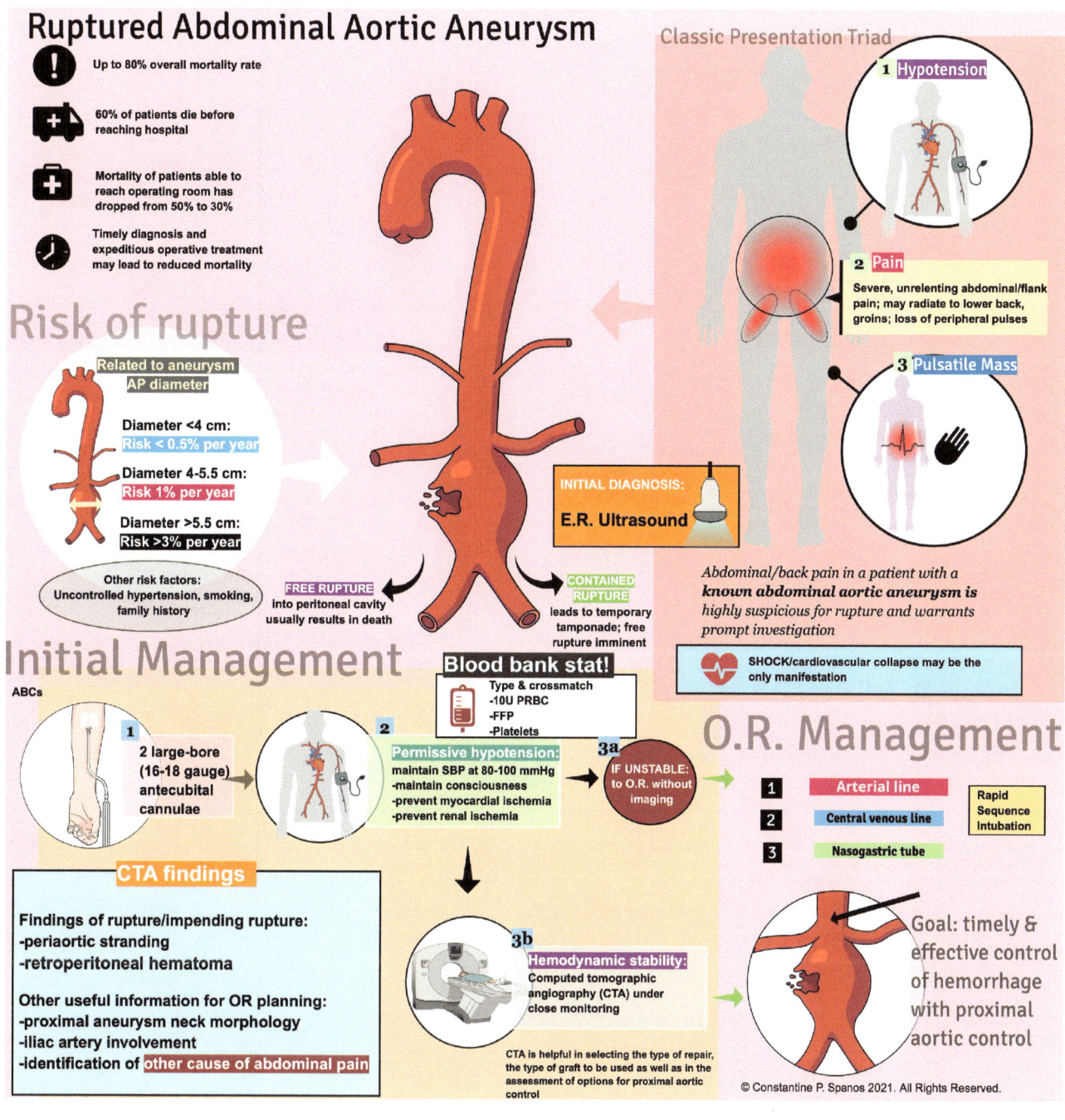

Up to 80% overall mortality rate

60% of patients die before reaching hospital

Mortality of patients able to reach operating room has dropped from 50% to 30%

Timely diagnosis and expeditious operative treatment may lead to reduced mortality

Risk of rupture

Related to aneurysm AP diameter

Diameter <4 cm:
Risk < 0.5% per year

Diameter 4-5.5 cm:
Risk 1% per year

Diameter >5.5 cm:
Risk >3% per year

Other risk factors:
Uncontrolled hypertension, smoking, family history

FREE RUPTURE into peritoneal cavity usually results in death

CONTAINED RUPTURE leads to temporary tamponade; free rupture imminent

Classic Presentation Triad

1 Hypotension

2 Pain
Severe, unrelenting abdominal/flank pain; may radiate to lower back, groins; loss of peripheral pulses

3 Pulsatile Mass

INITIAL DIAGNOSIS:
E.R. Ultrasound

Abdominal/back pain in a patient with a **known abdominal aortic aneurysm is** *highly suspicious for rupture and warrants prompt investigation*

SHOCK/cardiovascular collapse may be the only manifestation

Initial Management

ABCs

1 2 large-bore (16-18 gauge) antecubital cannulae

Blood bank stat!
Type & crossmatch
-10U PRBC
-FFP
-Platelets

2 **Permissive hypotension:** maintain SBP at 80-100 mmHg
-maintain consciousness
-prevent myocardial ischemia
-prevent renal ischemia

3a IF UNSTABLE: to O.R. without imaging

3b **Hemodynamic stability:** Computed tomographic angiography (CTA) under close monitoring

CTA is helpful in selecting the type of repair, the type of graft to be used as well as in the assessment of options for proximal aortic control

CTA findings

Findings of rupture/impending rupture:
-periaortic stranding
-retroperitoneal hematoma

Other useful information for OR planning:
-proximal aneurysm neck morphology
-iliac artery involvement
-identification of **other cause of abdominal pain**

O.R. Management

1 Arterial line

2 Central venous line

3 Nasogastric tube

Rapid Sequence Intubation

Goal: timely & effective control of hemorrhage with proximal aortic control

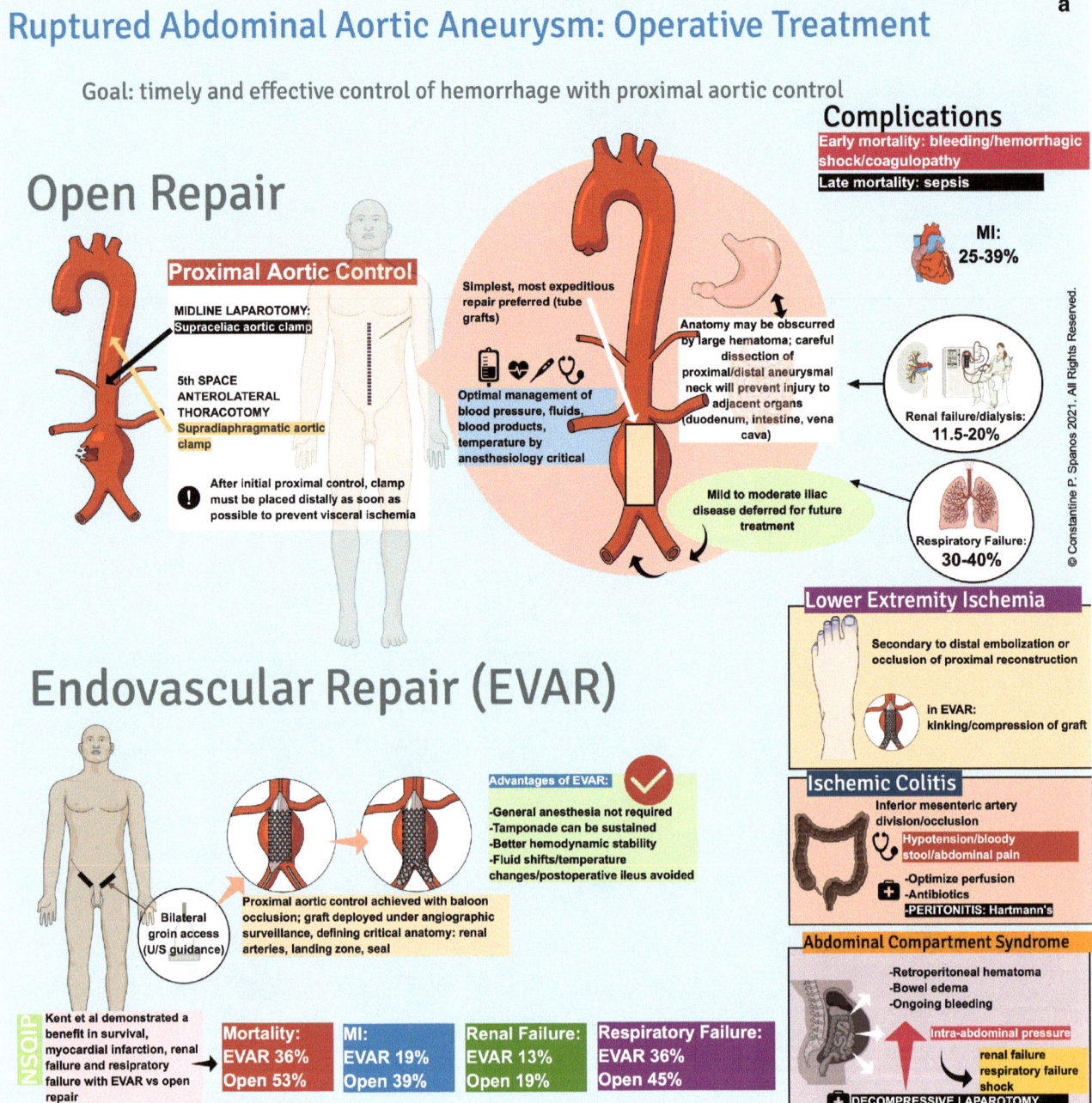

Ruptured Abdominal Aortic Aneurysm: Operative Treatment

Goal: timely and effective control of hemorrhage with proximal aortic control

a

Open Repair

Proximal Aortic Control

MIDLINE LAPAROTOMY:
Supraceliac aortic clamp

5th SPACE ANTEROLATERAL THORACOTOMY
Supradiaphragmatic aortic clamp

(!) After initial proximal control, clamp must be placed distally as soon as possible to prevent visceral ischemia

Simplest, most expeditious repair preferred (tube grafts)

Optimal management of blood pressure, fluids, blood products, temperature by anesthesiology critical

Anatomy may be obscured by large hematoma; careful dissection of proximal/distal aneurysmal neck will prevent injury to adjacent organs (duodenum, intestine, vena cava)

Mild to moderate iliac disease deferred for future treatment

Complications
Early mortality: bleeding/hemorrhagic shock/coagulopathy
Late mortality: sepsis

MI: 25-39%

Renal failure/dialysis: 11.5-20%

Respiratory Failure: 30-40%

Endovascular Repair (EVAR)

Bilateral groin access (U/S guidance)

Proximal aortic control achieved with baloon occlusion; graft deployed under angiographic surveillance, defining critical anatomy: renal arteries, landing zone, seal

Advantages of EVAR: ✓
-General anesthesia not required
-Tamponade can be sustained
-Better hemodynamic stability
-Fluid shifts/temperature changes/postoperative ileus avoided

NSQIP Kent et al demonstrated a benefit in survival, myocardial infarction, renal failure and respiratory failure with EVAR vs open repair →

Mortality:	**MI:**	**Renal Failure:**	**Respiratory Failure:**
EVAR 36%	EVAR 19%	EVAR 13%	EVAR 36%
Open 53%	Open 39%	Open 19%	Open 45%

Lower Extremity Ischemia
Secondary to distal embolization or occlusion of proximal reconstruction

in EVAR: kinking/compression of graft

Ischemic Colitis
Inferior mesenteric artery division/occlusion
Hypotension/bloody stool/abdominal pain
-Optimize perfusion
-Antibiotics
-PERITONITIS: Hartmann's

Abdominal Compartment Syndrome
-Retroperitoneal hematoma
-Bowel edema
-Ongoing bleeding

Intra-abdominal pressure
→ renal failure
respiratory failure
shock

DECOMPRESSIVE LAPAROTOMY

Ruptured Abdominal Aortic Aneurysm: Operative Treatment

b

Goal: timely and effective control of hemorrhage with proximal aortic control

Open Repair

Complications

Early mortality: bleeding/hemorrhagic shock/coagulopathy

Late mortality: sepsis

MI: 25-39%

Renal failure/dialysis: 11.5-20%

Respiratory Failure: 30-40%

Proximal Aortic Control

MIDLINE LAPAROTOMY:
Supraceliac aortic clamp

5th SPACE ANTEROLATERAL THORACOTOMY
Supradiaphragmatic aortic clamp

(!) After initial proximal control, clamp must be placed distally as soon as possible to prevent visceral ischemia

Simplest, most expeditious repair preferred (tube grafts)

Optimal management of blood pressure, fluids, blood products, temperature by anesthesiology critical

Anatomy may be obscured by large hematoma; careful dissection of proximal/distal aneurysmal neck will prevent injury to adjacent organs (duodenum, intestine, vena cava)

Mild to moderate iliac disease deferred for future treatment

© Constantine P.Spanos 2021. All Rights Reserved.

Lower Extremity Ischemia

Secondary to distal embolization or occlusion of proximal reconstruction

In EVAR: kinking/compression of graft

Endovascular Repair (EVAR)

Bilateral groin access (U/S guidance)

Proximal aortic control achieved with baloon occlusion; graft deployed under angiographic surveillance, defining critical anatomy: renal arteries, landing zone, seal

Advantages of EVAR: ✓

-General anesthesia not required
-Tamponade can be sustained
-Better hemodynamic stability
-Fluid shifts/temperature changes/postoperative ileus avoided

NSQIP Kent et al demonstrated a benefit in survival, myocardial infarction, renal failure and resipratory failure with EVAR vs open repair

Ischemic Colitis

Inferior mesenteric artery division/occlusion

Hypotension/bloody stool/abdominal pain

-Optimize perfusion
-Antibiotics
-PERITONITIS: Hartmann's

Abdominal Compartment Syndrome

-Retroperitoneal hematoma
-Bowel edema
-Ongoing bleeding

Intra-abdominal pressure

renal failure
respiratory failure
shock

DECOMPRESSIVE LAPAROTOMY

Mortality	MI	Renal Failure	Respiratory Failure
EVAR 36% / Open 53%	EVAR 19% / Open 39%	EVAR 13% / Open 19%	EVAR 36% / Open 45%

Further Reading

Chaikof EL, Brewster DC, Dalman RL, et al. The care of patients with an abdominal aortic aneurysm: the society for vascular surgery practice guidelines. J Vasc Surg. 2012;50(suppl 4):S2–S49.

Phelan PJ, Kent KC. The management of ruptured aortic aneurysm. In: Cameron JL, Cameron AM, editors. Current surgical therapy. 12th ed. Philadelphia: Elsevier; 2017. p. 916–21.

- Aortic dissection is a highly lethal vascular emergency. Without treatment, the mortality rate is 90%. This may drop to 20–25% if treated expeditiously. The incidence is 2.5–3.5 patients/100,000 per year. Aortic dissection is more frequent in elderly (60–80 year) males.
- Risk factors include hypertension, high-intensity weight lifting, presence of an aortic aneurysm, Marfan's/Ehler-Danlos/Loeys-Dietz disease, bicuspid aortic valve, pregnancy/delivery, and vasculitis.
- Aortic dissection occurs with sudden disruption of the aortic intima. The dissection propagates proximally and distally within the aortic media. True vascular luminal collapse may occur.
- Two aortic dissection classification systems are used most frequently: DeBakey and Stanford.
- **The DeBakey classification** is based on the site of dissection origin:
  - Type I: Origin at ascending aorta includes aortic arch and descending aorta
  - Type II: origin at ascending aorta; confined to ascending aorta
  - Type IIIa: Origin distal to subclavian artery; limited to descending thoracic aorta
  - Type IIIb: origin distal to subclavian artery; extends below the diaphragm
- **The Stanford classification** is based on involvement or not of the ascending aorta:
  - Type A: origin at ascending aorta (DeBakey type I, II)
  - Type B: origin at subclavian artery (DeBakey type IIIa, IIIb)
- Stanford type A aortic dissections are the most common (60%).
- Complicated Stanford dissections include those with rupture, malperfusion, refractory pain, and uncontrolled hypertension.
- The classic clinical presentation of aortic dissection includes acute severe "ripping" chest pain, with radiation to the upper back between the scapulae. This may be similar to a massive myocardial infarction. Many patients present with cardiovascular collapse or sudden death secondary to cardiac tamponade, myocardial ischemia, exsanguination, and heart failure.
- A pulse deficit may be present (weakened/absent carotid/radial/femoral pulse ± asymmetrical pulses).
- Aortic regurgitation is a common sequela of aortic dissection. A diastolic decrescendo murmur is characteristic and occurs in 50–75% of Stanford Type A dissections.
- ECG changes may be observed if dissection involves the coronary ostia and may be similar to myocardial infarction.
- Focal neurological deficits may occur; stroke, altered sensorium, a Horner's syndrome, and paraplegia are not uncommon.
- Myocardial ischemia, mesenteric ischemia, and renal ischemia may occur.
- High-resolution contrast-enhanced CT angiography is instrumental in the assessment of the entire aorta, may detect malperfusion, and aid in surgical planning.
- Transesophageal echocardiogram may detect cardiac tamponade, cardiac valvular dysfunction, and cardiac wall-motion abnormalities.
- Patients require continuous invasive hemodynamic monitoring in an ICU setting (radial/femoral arterial line). Intubation may be required.
- IV β-blockers are given to keep the heart rate <60–70 and SBP <100–110 mmHg; additional vasodilators may be required. These drugs must be given with caution in patients with aortic regurgitation.
- Stanford Type A dissections are surgical emergencies. A total aortic arch replacement is performed in cases with complex intimal arch disruption, large arch aneurysms (>5 cm), and patients with connective tissue disorders. If the aortic valve is involved, composite aortic root replacement with coronary "button reimplantation" (Bentall pro-

C. P. Spanos, *Acute Surgical Topics*, https://doi.org/10.1007/978-3-030-68700-7_19

cedure) is performed. Cardiopulmonary bypass with circulatory arrest is utilized in these cases. The surgical mortality is 25–30%.

- Uncomplicated Stanford Type B dissections are treated medically, with heart rate and blood pressure control using β-blockers.

- Complicated Stanford B dissections can be treated with thoracic endovascular aortic repair (TEVAR) with 60–80% survival rates. Open surgical repair is fraught with high morbidity and mortality.

Aortic Dissection

Highly lethal vascular emergency; 90% mortality without treatment; 20-25% mortality with timely treatment

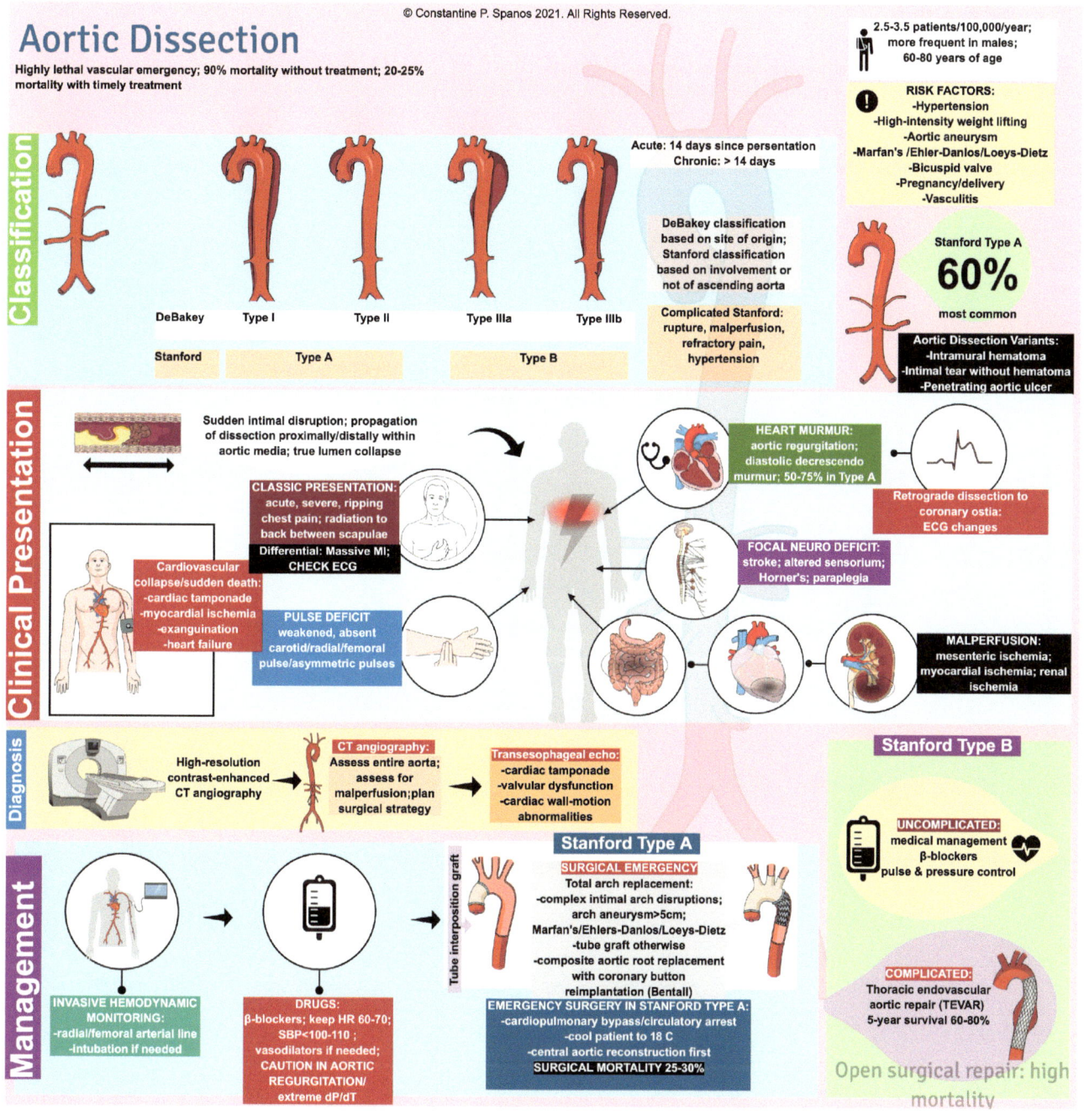

Classification

DeBakey   Type I   Type II   Type IIIa   Type IIIb

Stanford   Type A   Type B

Acute: 14 days since persentation
Chronic: > 14 days

DeBakey classification based on site of origin; Stanford classification based on involvement or not of ascending aorta

Complicated Stanford: rupture, malperfusion, refractory pain, hypertension

2.5-3.5 patients/100,000/year; more frequent in males; 60-80 years of age

RISK FACTORS:
-Hypertension
-High-intensity weight lifting
-Aortic aneurysm
-Marfan's /Ehler-Danlos/Loeys-Dietz
-Bicuspid valve
-Pregnancy/delivery
-Vasculitis

Stanford Type A
60%
most common

Aortic Dissection Variants:
-Intramural hematoma
-Intimal tear without hematoma
-Penetrating aortic ulcer

Clinical Presentation

Sudden intimal disruption; propagation of dissection proximally/distally within aortic media; true lumen collapse

CLASSIC PRESENTATION:
acute, severe, ripping chest pain; radiation to back between scapulae
Differential: Massive MI; CHECK ECG

Cardiovascular collapse/sudden death:
-cardiac tamponade
-myocardial ischemia
-exanguination
-heart failure

PULSE DEFICIT
weakened, absent carotid/radial/femoral pulse/asymmetric pulses

HEART MURMUR:
aortic regurgitation; diastolic decrescendo murmur; 50-75% in Type A

Retrograde dissection to coronary ostia: ECG changes

FOCAL NEURO DEFICIT:
stroke; altered sensorium; Horner's; paraplegia

MALPERFUSION:
mesenteric ischemia; myocardial ischemia; renal ischemia

Diagnosis

High-resolution contrast-enhanced CT angiography

CT angiography:
Assess entire aorta; assess for malperfusion;plan surgical strategy

Transesophageal echo:
-cardiac tamponade
-valvular dysfunction
-cardiac wall-motion abnormalities

Management

INVASIVE HEMODYNAMIC MONITORING:
-radial/femoral arterial line
-intubation if needed

DRUGS:
β-blockers; keep HR 60-70; SBP<100-110 ;
vasodilators if needed;
CAUTION IN AORTIC REGURGITATION/ extreme dP/dT

Tube interposition graft

Stanford Type A

SURGICAL EMERGENCY
Total arch replacement:
-complex intimal arch disruptions; arch aneurysm>5cm;
Marfan's/Ehlers-Danlos/Loeys-Dietz
-tube graft otherwise
-composite aortic root replacement with coronary button reimplantation (Bentall)

EMERGENCY SURGERY IN STANFORD TYPE A:
-cardiopulmonary bypass/circulatory arrest
-cool patient to 18 C
-central aortic reconstruction first
SURGICAL MORTALITY 25-30%

Stanford Type B

UNCOMPLICATED:
medical management
β-blockers
pulse & pressure control

COMPLICATED:
Thoracic endovascular aortic repair (TEVAR)
5-year survival 60-80%

Open surgical repair: high mortality

Further Reading

Isselbacher EM. Trends in thoracic aneurysms and dissection: out of the shadows and into the light. Circulation. 2014;130:2267–8.

Kim KM, MacGillivray TE. The management of acute aortic dissections. In: Cameron JL, Cameron AM, editors. Current surgical therapy. 12th ed. Philadelphia: Elsevier; 2017. p. 933–7.

- Peripheral arterial embolism is an acute vascular emergency which requires timely diagnosis and prompt therapeutic interventions. Delay in diagnosis leads to significantly increased morbidity, mortality, and limb loss.
- Most arterial emboli originate from the left atrium in patients with atrial fibrillation, or the left ventricle in patients with a recent history of myocardial infarction. Approximately 0.5% of patients with atrial fibrillation will suffer a non-cerebrovascular embolic event. Of these, 2/3 will occur in the extremities and 1/3 in the visceral mesenteric circulation.
- Other sources of emboli include:
  - Right atrial myxoma
  - Valvular heart disease (endocarditis, rheumatic fever)
  - Prosthetic heart valves
  - Atherosclerotic plaques
  - Vascular trauma
  - Deep venous thrombi; with paradoxical arterial embolism via atrial/ventricular septal defects
- The embolic material may consist of a thrombus, cholesterol, air, fat, tissue, amniotic fluid, or a foreign body.
- The majority of peripheral emboli occur in the lower extremity (84%). The upper extremity is involved in 16% of cases.
- Peripheral arterial embolism classically presents with the "6 P's": **pain, pulselessness, poikilothermia, pallor, paresthesia, and paralysis**. These are the hallmarks of acute ischemia, without established collateral circulation. The onset of symptoms is rapid.
- A history of claudication (occurring for weeks and months), as well as rest pain, points to a diagnosis of acute thrombosis of progressive atherosclerotic peripheral arterial disease, rather than acute embolism. Of note, these patients often have established collateral circulation.
- Back pain may be suggestive of acute aortic dissection, which must be ruled out. In addition, aneurysmal disease (aortic, iliac, popliteal) must also be excluded.

- On physical exam, the affected and unaffected extremity must be compared. The most common findings include:
  - Pallor, livedo reticularis, or cyanotic mottling
  - Absent pulses or Doppler signals
  - Absent capillary refill
  - "Water hammer" pulse proximal to embolic obstruction
  - Diminished sensation (first web-space in dorsal foot)
  - Weakness in dorsiflexion (peroneal nerve)
- It is important to classify the degree of limb ischemia into nonthreatening, threatened, or irreversible. This may guide the diagnostic and therapeutic maneuvers appropriate for each patient.
- Many patients with acute peripheral embolism have a significantly increased cardiovascular risk profile. Post-intervention cardiovascular complications are frequent.
- Do not delay intervention/treatment to obtain a precise diagnosis with imaging; institutional logistics and availability may cause undue delays. Limb loss and ischemia-reperfusion syndrome should always be taken into account.
- Available imaging modalities include duplex ultrasound, CT angiography, MR angiography, and conventional angiography.
- The goal in managing peripheral arterial embolism is to restore blood flow to the extremity prior to the onset of irreversible tissue damage. In addition, reperfusion injury and further limb ischemia must be prevented, diagnosed, and treated.
- The initial management strategy includes resuscitation (with IV fluids) and anticoagulation with either unfractionated heparin or therapeutic doses of low molecular weight heparin. The aPTT must be maintained at a level of 60–80 sec. Avoid the use of potassium in IV fluids, as reperfusion may result in significant hyperkalemia.
- A basic metabolic panel, CBC, PT/PTT, CPK, and lactate are obtained, as well as blood type and screen.
- Renal toxicity may be avoided and/or treated with mannitol diuresis and bicarbonate infusion (with a goal of urine alkalinization).

- Restoration of extremity blood can be achieved with surgical thromboembolectomy and percutaneous vascular techniques. The latter include catheter-directed pharmacological thrombolysis, percutaneous mechanical thrombectomy.
- Time to reperfusion is critical. **The ideal time to reperfusion is within 6 h**. Restoration of blood flow more than 6 h after embolic event runs the risk of compartment syndrome.
- Surgical thromboembolectomy is performed by accessing both femoral vessels in the case of lower extremity embolism and the brachial artery in upper extremity embolism. Inflatable Fogarty catheters are the mainstay of surgical intervention. The catheters are advanced proximally and distally; the goal is to restore prograde flow and clear distal circulation. There is a risk of further embolization with either clot and/or atheromatous material; in upper extremity interventions, there is a risk of cerebrovascular embolism.
- Reperfusion is assessed with Doppler interrogation and on-table angiography.
- Catheter-directed thrombolysis utilizes tPA, streptokinase, or urokinase (lytic agents). Arteriography is used to localize the thrombus. A catheter guidewire transverses the thrombus and the lytic agent is infused into the thrombus.
- Percutaneous mechanical thrombectomy uses suction, rotational infusion, ultrasound, or a high-velocity rheolytic jet to dissolute the clot and expose it to lytic agents thus facilitating lysis.
- Thrombolysis is associated with higher rates of stroke, major bleeding, and distal embolization. It is optimal for small-vessel embolization, through which Fogarty catheters would not be able to pass.

- Contraindications to thrombolysis include active bleeding, stroke, trauma, intracranial tumors, surgery within 3 months of embolism, end-stage liver disease, active peptic ulcer disease, and coagulopathy.
- Post-procedure management includes hemodynamic monitoring, careful consideration of acid/base balance, and electrolyte abnormalities. Delay in blood flow restoration increases the incidence of acute extremity compartment syndrome. Fasciotomies should be performed either prophylactically or after confirmation of abnormal extremity compartment pressures.
- Ischemia/reperfusion syndrome may occur when toxic metabolites are released into the systemic circulation. Rhabdomyolysis may induce acute tubular necrosis and renal failure. Infusion of bicarbonate and mannitol may facilitate myoglobin renal excretion. Multi-organ system failure is a deleterious sequela of ischemia/reperfusion syndrome.
- In class III (irreversible) limb ischemia, amputation may be necessary. Revascularization in this instance may lead to profound ischemia/reperfusion syndrome.
- After intervention, anticoagulation must be continued. Initially, heparin is administered. This can be replaced by direct thrombin inhibitors (lepirudin/argatroban) with subsequent transition to oral anticoagulation.
- In most cases of acute peripheral artery embolism, emergent treatment is performed prior to investigation of the underlying etiology. Investigation includes:
  - Transesophageal echocardiography (detection of valvular vegetations, cardiac chamber thrombi, shunts)
  - CT angiogram of chest, abdomen, pelvis (detection of AAA, arterial ulceration, intimal flap, atherosclerotic lesion, thrombus)
  - Hypercoagulability workup
  - DVT assessment (paradoxical embolization)

Peripheral Arterial Embolism

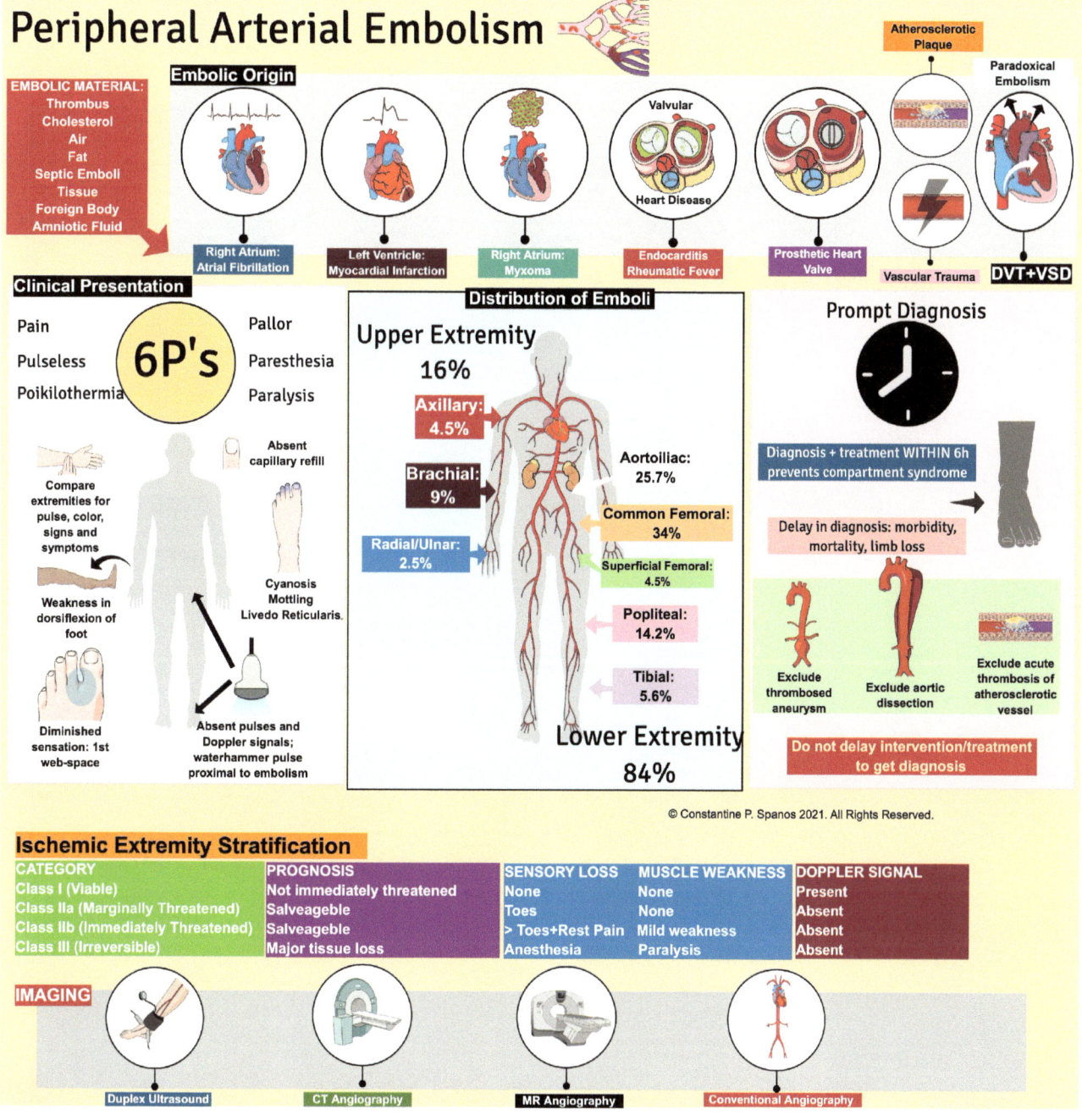

Embolic Origin

EMBOLIC MATERIAL:
Thrombus
Cholesterol
Air
Fat
Septic Emboli
Tissue
Foreign Body
Amniotic Fluid

Atherosclerotic Plaque

Paradoxical Embolism

Valvular

Heart Disease

Right Atrium: Atrial Fibrillation
Left Ventricle: Myocardial Infarction
Right Atrium: Myxoma
Endocarditis Rheumatic Fever
Prosthetic Heart Valve
Vascular Trauma
DVT+VSD

Clinical Presentation

Pain — Pallor
Pulseless — Paresthesia
Poikilothermia — Paralysis

6P's

Compare extremities for pulse, color, signs and symptoms

Weakness in dorsiflexion of foot

Diminished sensation: 1st web-space

Absent capillary refill

Cyanosis Mottling Livedo Reticularis.

Absent pulses and Doppler signals; waterhammer pulse proximal to embolism

Distribution of Emboli

Upper Extremity 16%

Axillary: 4.5%
Brachial: 9%
Radial/Ulnar: 2.5%

Aortoiliac: 25.7%
Common Femoral: 34%
Superficial Femoral: 4.5%
Popliteal: 14.2%
Tibial: 5.6%

Lower Extremity 84%

Prompt Diagnosis

Diagnosis + treatment WITHIN 6h prevents compartment syndrome

Delay in diagnosis: morbidity, mortality, limb loss

Exclude thrombosed aneurysm
Exclude aortic dissection
Exclude acute thrombosis of atherosclerotic vessel

Do not delay intervention/treatment to get diagnosis

Ischemic Extremity Stratification

CATEGORY	PROGNOSIS	SENSORY LOSS	MUSCLE WEAKNESS	DOPPLER SIGNAL
Class I (Viable)	Not immediately threatened	None	None	Present
Class IIa (Marginally Threatened)	Salveageble	Toes	None	Absent
Class IIb (Immediately Threatened)	Salveageble	> Toes+Rest Pain	Mild weakness	Absent
Class III (Irreversible)	Major tissue loss	Anesthesia	Paralysis	Absent

IMAGING

Duplex Ultrasound — CT Angiography — MR Angiography — Conventional Angiography

Peripheral Arterial Embolism: Management

Goal is to restore blood flow to extremity prior to onset of irreversible tissue damage, thus preventing limb loss and reducing morbidity & mortality

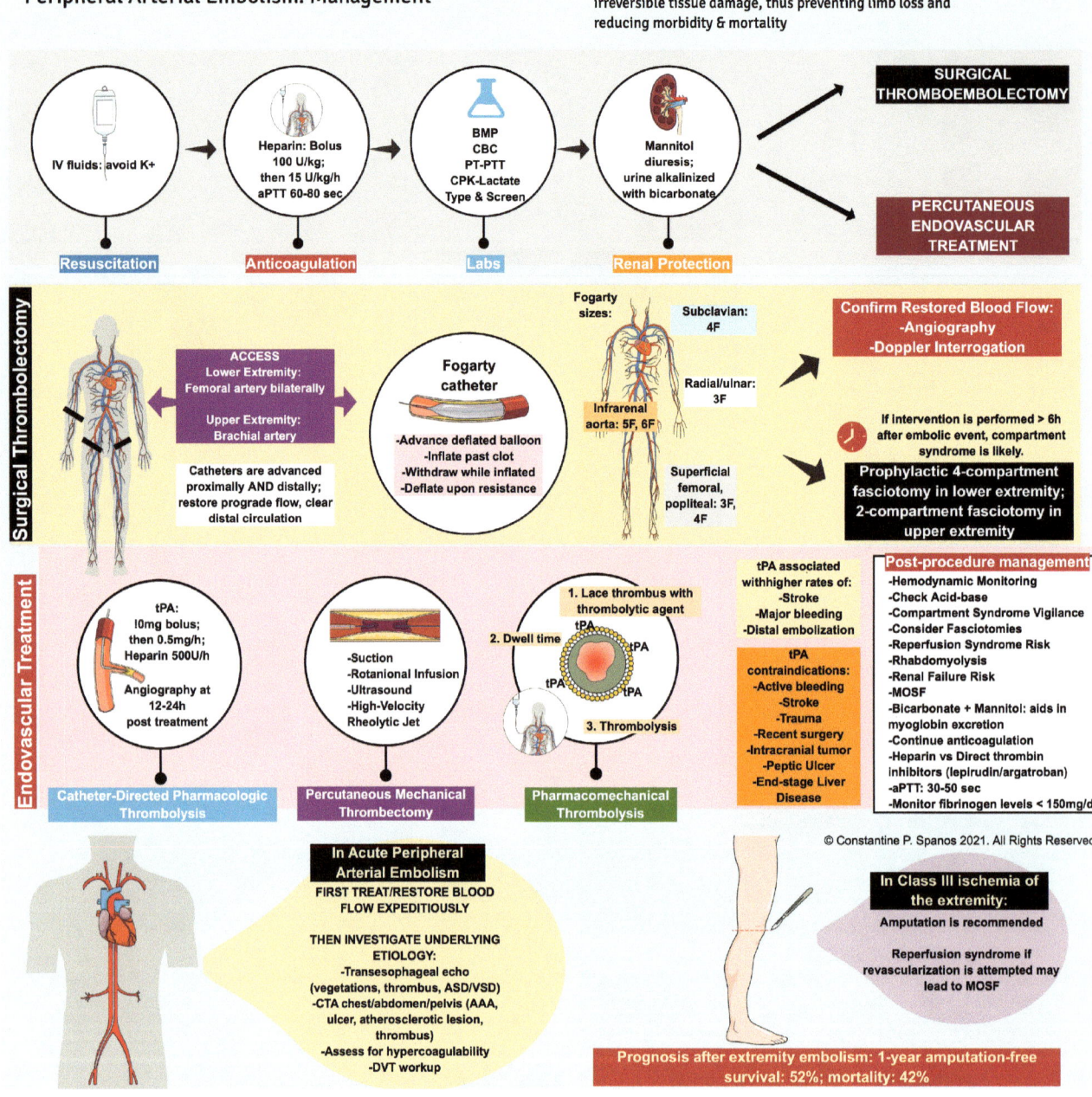

Resuscitation — IV fluids: avoid K+

Anticoagulation — Heparin: Bolus 100 U/kg; then 15 U/kg/h aPTT 60-80 sec

Labs — BMP, CBC, PT-PTT, CPK-Lactate, Type & Screen

Renal Protection — Mannitol diuresis; urine alkalinized with bicarbonate

SURGICAL THROMBOEMBOLECTOMY

PERCUTANEOUS ENDOVASCULAR TREATMENT

Surgical Thrombolectomy

ACCESS
Lower Extremity: Femoral artery bilaterally
Upper Extremity: Brachial artery

Catheters are advanced proximally AND distally; restore prograde flow, clear distal circulation

Fogarty catheter
-Advance deflated balloon
-Inflate past clot
-Withdraw while inflated
-Deflate upon resistance

Fogarty sizes:
Infrarenal aorta: 5F, 6F
Subclavian: 4F
Radial/ulnar: 3F
Superficial femoral, popliteal: 3F, 4F

Confirm Restored Blood Flow:
-Angiography
-Doppler Interrogation

If intervention is performed > 6h after embolic event, compartment syndrome is likely.

Prophylactic 4-compartment fasciotomy in lower extremity; 2-compartment fasciotomy in upper extremity

Endovascular Treatment

Catheter-Directed Pharmacologic Thrombolysis
tPA: 10mg bolus; then 0.5mg/h; Heparin 500U/h
Angiography at 12-24h post treatment

Percutaneous Mechanical Thrombectomy
-Suction
-Rotational Infusion
-Ultrasound
-High-Velocity Rheolytic Jet

Pharmacomechanical Thrombolysis
1. Lace thrombus with thrombolytic agent tPA
2. Dwell time
3. Thrombolysis

tPA associated with higher rates of:
-Stroke
-Major bleeding
-Distal embolization

tPA contraindications:
-Active bleeding
-Stroke
-Trauma
-Recent surgery
-Intracranial tumor
-Peptic Ulcer
-End-stage Liver Disease

Post-procedure management
-Hemodynamic Monitoring
-Check Acid-base
-Compartment Syndrome Vigilance
-Consider Fasciotomies
-Reperfusion Syndrome Risk
-Rhabdomyolysis
-Renal Failure Risk
-MOSF
-Bicarbonate + Mannitol: aids in myoglobin excretion
-Continue anticoagulation
-Heparin vs Direct thrombin inhibitors (lepirudin/argatroban)
-aPTT: 30-50 sec
-Monitor fibrinogen levels < 150mg/dl

In Acute Peripheral Arterial Embolism
FIRST TREAT/RESTORE BLOOD FLOW EXPEDITIOUSLY

THEN INVESTIGATE UNDERLYING ETIOLOGY:
-Transesophageal echo (vegetations, thrombus, ASD/VSD)
-CTA chest/abdomen/pelvis (AAA, ulcer, atherosclerotic lesion, thrombus)
-Assess for hypercoagulability
-DVT workup

In Class III ischemia of the extremity:
Amputation is recommended

Reperfusion syndrome if revascularization is attempted may lead to MOSF

Prognosis after extremity embolism: 1-year amputation-free survival: 52%; mortality: 42%

Further Reading

Berridge DC, Kessel DO, Robertson I. Surgery versus thrombolysis for initial management of acute limb ischemia. Cochrane Database Syst Rev. 2013;2013(6):CD002784.

Leung DA, Blitz LR, Nelson T, et al. Rheolytic pharmacomechanical thrombectomy for the management of acute limb ischemia: results from the PEARL registry. J Endovasc Ther. 2015;22:546–57.

Patel MS, Chaikof EL. Peripheral arterial embolism. In: Cameron JL, Cameron AM, editors. Current surgical therapy. 12th ed. Philadelphia: Elsevier; 2017. p. 1031–324.

Rutherford RB, Baker JD, Ernst C, et al. Recommended standards for reports dealing with lower extremity ischemia: revised version. J Vasc Surg. 1997;26:517–38.

- Hypercoagulable states are usually diagnosed **after** a venous thromboembolic episode (VTE). Examples of VTE include deep venous thrombosis, pulmonary embolism (PE). Multiple spontaneous abortions should raise suspicion of hypercoagulability as well.
- Hypercoagulability can be acquired (provoked) or inherited (unprovoked). **Virchow's triad** (stasis, endothelial injury, increased platelets) contributes to pathological thrombosis.
- Risk factors for provoked hypercoagulability include:
  - Recent surgery
  - Immobility
  - Trauma
  - Cancer
  - Contraceptive drugs/hormone replacement therapy/ testosterone therapy
- Inherited hypercoagulability is usually secondary to a genetic mutation. The most common mutation is in factor V (Leiden). This causes hypercoagulability through resistance to activated protein C. It can be diagnosed with a functional activated protein C assay or detection of the mutation with genetic testing. Other inherited causes of hypercoagulability include prothrombin G20210 mutation, protein C/S deficiency, antiphospholipid syndrome, and antithrombin deficiency.
- Patients with DVT present with swelling, pain, warmth, and tenderness in an extremity. In severe cases, there may be a loss of pedal pulses.
- Patients with PE present with tachypnea, dyspnea, tachycardia. The ECG may depict right heart strain, inverted T waves in the right precordial leads. ABG may show hypoxemia and hypocapnia.
- Diagnostic of DVT is achieved with duplex ultrasound; CT angiogram is the standard exam for PE. A negative D-Dimer test virtually excludes VTE.

- The **Wells Clinical Pretest Probability Score** for DVT can estimate risk for DVT with relative accuracy.
- Heparin-induced thrombocytopenia occurs after prior exposure to heparin. Antibodies to the PF4 complex induce a hypercoagulable state and may cause both venous and arterial thrombosis. A platelet reduction of 50% from baseline is highly suspicious of HIT. An anti-PF4 antibody assay confirms the diagnosis. Treatment is initiated before lab confirmation by removing all sources of heparin and administration of direct thrombin inhibitors (bivalirudin, argatroban) or direct factor Xa inhibition (fondaparinux).
- VTE is initially treated with unfractionated heparin infusion with transition to oral anticoagulants after therapeutic levels of heparin dosing have been achieved. Alternatively, low molecular weight heparin, given subcutaneously, can be given. Duration of anticoagulation therapy is usually 3 months for provoked hypercoagulability, and 6 months for unprovoked hypercoagulability.
- Extension of anticoagulation therapy beyond 6 months should be considered in:
  - Unprovoked symptomatic VTE
  - Recurrent unprovoked VTE
  - Active malignancy after VTE
  - Inherited protein C/s deficiency
  - Homozygous factor V/Leiden mutation
  - Other homozygous mutations
- The **Vienna Prediction Model** uses sex, VTE location, D-dimer levels to assess the risk of recurrence, and need for continuation of anticoagulation therapy.

C. P. Spanos, *Acute Surgical Topics*, https://doi.org/10.1007/978-3-030-68700-7_21

Hypercoagulability

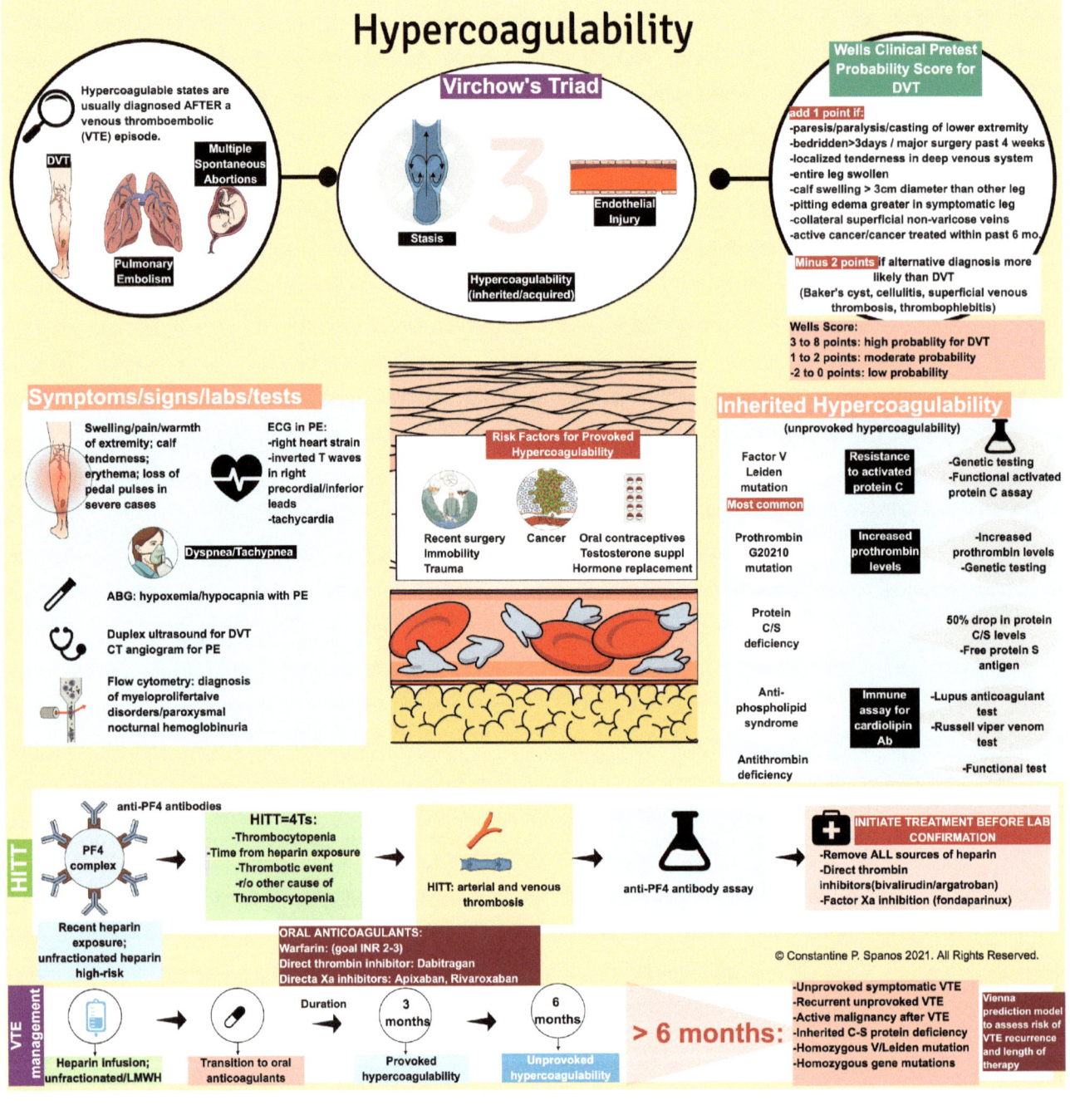

Hypercoagulable states are usually diagnosed AFTER a venous thromboembolism (VTE) episode.

DVT

Multiple Spontaneous Abortions

Pulmonary Embolism

Virchow's Triad

3

Stasis

Endothelial Injury

Hypercoagulability (inherited/acquired)

Wells Clinical Pretest Probability Score for DVT

add 1 point if:
-paresis/paralysis/casting of lower extremity
-bedridden>3days / major surgery past 4 weeks
-localized tenderness in deep venous system
-entire leg swollen
-calf swelling > 3cm diameter than other leg
-pitting edema greater in symptomatic leg
-collateral superficial non-varicose veins
-active cancer/cancer treated within past 6 mo.

Minus 2 points if alternative diagnosis more likely than DVT
(Baker's cyst, cellulitis, superficial venous thrombosis, thrombophlebitis)

Wells Score:
3 to 8 points: high probability for DVT
1 to 2 points: moderate probability
-2 to 0 points: low probability

Symptoms/signs/labs/tests

Swelling/pain/warmth of extremity; calf tenderness; erythema; loss of pedal pulses in severe cases

ECG in PE:
-right heart strain
-inverted T waves in right precordial/inferior leads
-tachycardia

Dyspnea/Tachypnea

ABG: hypoxemia/hypocapnia with PE

Duplex ultrasound for DVT
CT angiogram for PE

Flow cytometry: diagnosis of myeloprolifertaive disorders/paroxysmal nocturnal hemoglobinuria

Risk Factors for Provoked Hypercoagulability

Recent surgery
Immobility
Trauma

Cancer

Oral contraceptives
Testosterone suppl
Hormone replacement

Inherited Hypercoagulability
(unprovoked hypercoagulability)

Factor V Leiden mutation **Most common**	Resistance to activated protein C	-Genetic testing -Functional activated protein C assay
Prothrombin G20210 mutation	Increased prothrombin levels	-Increased prothrombin levels -Genetic testing
Protein C/S deficiency		50% drop in protein C/S levels -Free protein S antigen
Anti-phospholipid syndrome	Immune assay for cardiolipin Ab	-Lupus anticoagulant test -Russell viper venom test
Antithrombin deficiency		-Functional test

HITT

anti-PF4 antibodies

PF4 complex

HITT=4Ts:
-Thrombocytopenia
-Time from heparin exposure
-Thrombotic event
-r/o other cause of Thrombocytopenia

HITT: arterial and venous thrombosis

anti-PF4 antibody assay

INITIATE TREATMENT BEFORE LAB CONFIRMATION
-Remove ALL sources of heparin
-Direct thrombin inhibitors(bivalirudin/argatroban)
-Factor Xa inhibition (fondaparinux)

Recent heparin exposure; unfractionated heparin high-risk

ORAL ANTICOAGULANTS:
Warfarin: (goal INR 2-3)
Direct thrombin inhibitor: Dabitragan
Directa Xa inhibitors: Apixaban, Rivaroxaban

VTE management

Heparin infusion; unfractionated/LMWH

Transition to oral anticoagulants

Duration

3 months
Provoked hypercoagulability

6 months
Unprovoked hypercoagulability

> 6 months:
-Unprovoked symptomatic VTE
-Recurrent unprovoked VTE
-Active malignancy after VTE
-Inherited C-S protein deficiency
-Homozygous V/Leiden mutation
-Homozygous gene mutations

Vienna prediction model to assess risk of VTE recurrence and length of therapy

Further Reading

Arepally GM, Ortel TL. Heparin-induced thrombocytopenia. N Engl J Med. 2006;355:809–17.

Ehlert BA. Hypercoagulable patient. In: McIntyre Jr RC, Schulick RD, editors. Surgical decision making. 6th ed. Philadelphia: Elsevier; 2020. p. 14–5.

Eichinger S, Heinze G, Jandeck LM, et al. Risk assessment of recurrence in patients with unprovoked deep vein thrombosis or pulmonary embolism: the Vienna Prediction Model. Circulation. 2010;121:1630–6.

- Asepsis, hemostasis, and gentle handling of tissues are principle tenets of surgery. Hemostasis may be affected by bleeding disorders. A careful history and physical exam are the first steps in detecting bleeding/coagulation abnormalities.
- Bleeding disorders are highly suspected when a patient reports the following:
  - Significant bleeding after surgery, endoscopy, and dental procedures
  - Easy bruising, skin petechiae
  - Heavy menstrual flow
  - Hemarthrosis
  - Epistaxis
  - History of renal disease, hepatic disease, leukemia, and autoimmune disorders
- Medications that cause increased bleeding tendency include antiplatelet and anticoagulant drugs.
- A CBC will provide a gross estimate of circulating cellular blood components.
- Platelet counts of <20,000 may be associated with spontaneous bleeding
- Platelet dysfunction is not uncommon in dialysis patients.
- Elevated INR is a result of coumadin and/or hepatic disease.
- Elevated PTT is a result of unfractionated heparin administration
- Low fibrinogen levels are the result of massive bleeding, blood component consumption or dilution, acidosis, and hyperfibrinolysis. The Clauss fibrinogen assay is used as a guide for treatment.
- D-dimer levels measure fibrinolysis degradation products. As a rule of thumb, increased D-dimer levels combined with decreased fibrinogen levels denote disseminated intravascular coagulation (DIC).
- Thromboelastography can provide a broad functional assessment of the coagulation system, and guide blood component therapy. The following parameters are key:
  - R: period of latency until initial fibrin formation. Represents enzymatic portion of coagulation.
  - K: Speed to reach a certain level of clot strength. Represents clot kinetics.
  - α: Represents fibrinogen level.
  - MA: Maximum amplitude. Represents platelet aggregation/function.
  - LY30: Rate of amplitude reduction after 30 min. Represents clot lysis.
- Bleeding associated with hepatic disease can be treated with vitamin K, prothrombin complex concentrate (PCC), FFP, and cryoprecipitate.
- Severe sepsis and massive obstetric bleeding are causes of DIC. The underlying condition must be treated; platelets are transfused when <50,000; cryoprecipitate when fibrinogen <100 mg/dl.
- Cryoprecipitate, tranexamic acid, aminocaproic acid reduces surgical bleeding in cardiothoracic, orthopedic, and high-risk obstetrical surgery. Tranexamic acid administration confers an increased risk of thrombosis.
- In trauma-induced coagulopathy, component-directed therapy using thromboelastography may be optimal.
- Warfarin/Coumadin is reversed by vitamin K, FFP, and prothrombin complex concentrate (PCC).
- Direct oral anticoagulants are reversed as follows:
  - Dabitragan: idarucizumab
  - Apixaban/rivaroxaban: andexanet-α, PCC
- Patients with hemophilia A and B may be treated with factor concentrates when they are available. FFP can be used alternatively.
- Patients with von Willebrand disease type I and II are treated with DDAVP. Patients with von Willebrand type III are treated with von Willebrand factor or cryoprecipitate and/or FFP.
- Platelet dysfunction with bleeding tendency is common in renal dialysis patients. Treatment is possible with administration of DDAVP, cryoprecipitate. Bleeding uremic patients are treated with dialysis.

Bleeding Disorders

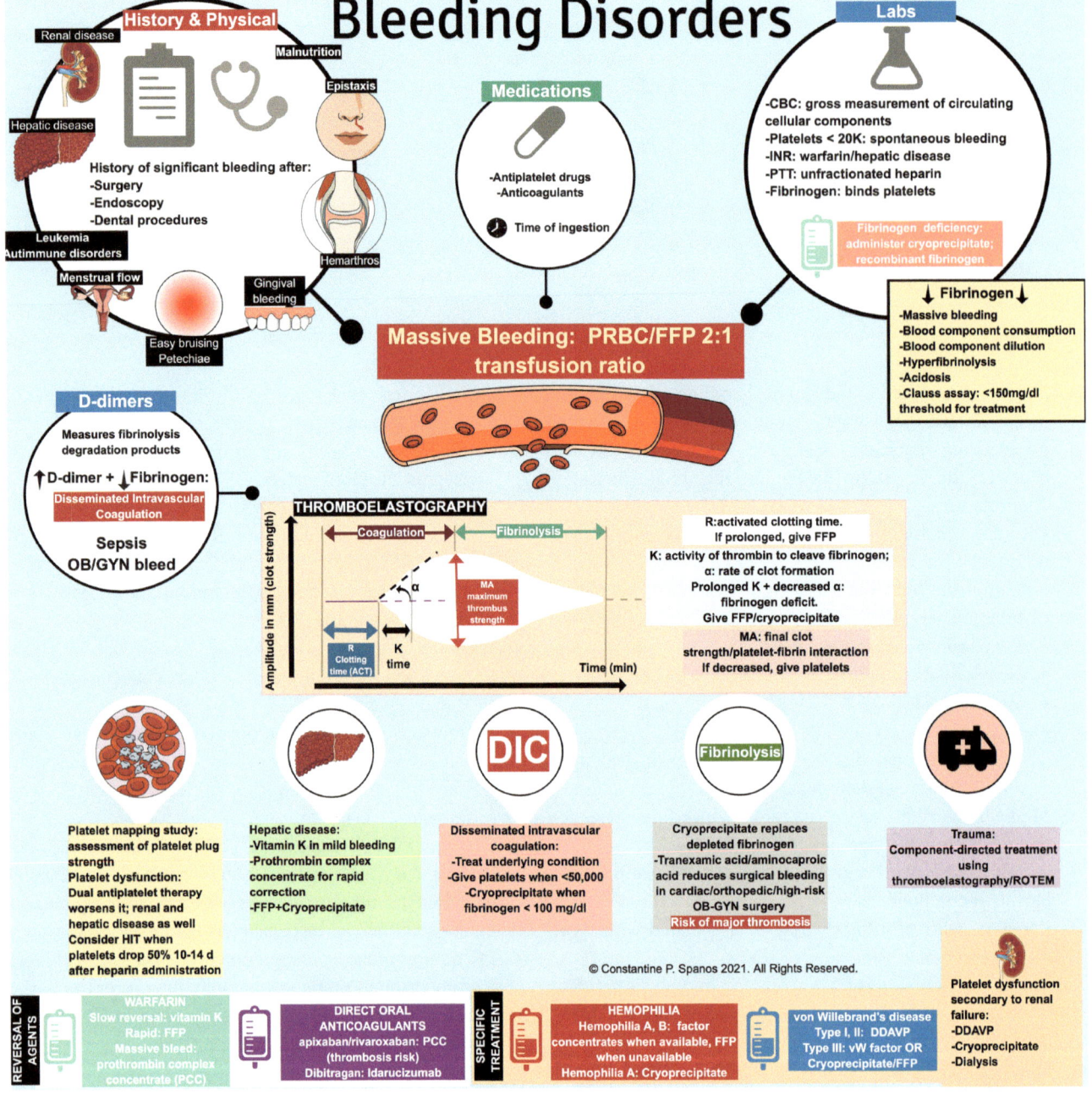

History & Physical

Renal disease

Malnutrition

Epistaxis

Hepatic disease

History of significant bleeding after:
-Surgery
-Endoscopy
-Dental procedures

Leukemia
Autimmune disorders

Hemarthros

Menstrual flow

Gingival bleeding

Easy bruising
Petechiae

Medications

-Antiplatelet drugs
-Anticoagulants

Time of ingestion

Labs

-CBC: gross measurement of circulating cellular components
-Platelets < 20K: spontaneous bleeding
-INR: warfarin/hepatic disease
-PTT: unfractionated heparin
-Fibrinogen: binds platelets

Fibrinogen deficiency: administer cryoprecipitate; recombinant fibrinogen

↓ Fibrinogen ↓
-Massive bleeding
-Blood component consumption
-Blood component dilution
-Hyperfibrinolysis
-Acidosis
-Clauss assay: <150mg/dl threshold for treatment

Massive Bleeding: PRBC/FFP 2:1 transfusion ratio

D-dimers

Measures fibrinolysis degradation products

↑D-dimer + ↓Fibrinogen:
Disseminated Intravascular Coagulation

Sepsis
OB/GYN bleed

THROMBOELASTOGRAPHY

Coagulation   Fibrinolysis

Amplitude in mm (clot strength)

α

MA maximum thrombus strength

R Clotting time (ACT)   K time

Time (min)

R:activated clotting time.
If prolonged, give FFP
K: activity of thrombin to cleave fibrinogen;
α: rate of clot formation
Prolonged K + decreased α:
fibrinogen deficit.
Give FFP/cryoprecipitate
MA: final clot
strength/platelet-fibrin interaction
If decreased, give platelets

Platelet mapping study: assessment of platelet plug strength
Platelet dysfunction:
Dual antiplatelet therapy worsens it; renal and hepatic disease as well
Consider HIT when platelets drop 50% 10-14 d after heparin administration

Hepatic disease:
-Vitamin K in mild bleeding
-Prothrombin complex concentrate for rapid correction
-FFP+Cryoprecipitate

DIC

Disseminated intravascular coagulation:
-Treat underlying condition
-Give platelets when <50,000
-Cryoprecipitate when fibrinogen < 100 mg/dl

Fibrinolysis

Cryoprecipitate replaces depleted fibrinogen
-Tranexamic acid/aminocaproic acid reduces surgical bleeding in cardiac/orthopedic/high-risk OB-GYN surgery
Risk of major thrombosis

Trauma:
Component-directed treatment using thromboelastography/ROTEM

© Constantine P. Spanos 2021. All Rights Reserved.

Platelet dysfunction secondary to renal failure:
-DDAVP
-Cryoprecipitate
-Dialysis

REVERSAL OF AGENTS

WARFARIN
Slow reversal: vitamin K
Rapid: FFP
Massive bleed: prothrombin complex concentrate (PCC)

DIRECT ORAL ANTICOAGULANTS
apixaban/rivaroxaban: PCC (thrombosis risk)
Dibitragan: Idarucizumab

SPECIFIC TREATMENT

HEMOPHILIA
Hemophilia A, B: factor concentrates when available, FFP when unavailable
Hemophilia A: Cryoprecipitate

von Willebrand's disease
Type I, II: DDAVP
Type III: vW factor OR Cryoprecipitate/FFP

Further Reading

Gonzalez E, Moore EE, Moore HB. Management of trauma-induced coagulopathy with thromboelastography. Crit Care Clin. 2017;33:119–34.

Samuels JM, Morre HB, Moore EE. Bleeding disorders in surgical patients. In: McIntyre Jr RC, Schulick RD, editors. Surgical decision making. 6th ed. Philadelphia: Elsevier; 2020. p. 10–2.